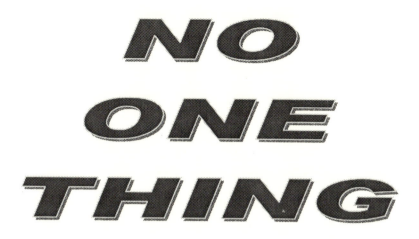

NO ONE THING

To Master Your Life

THE ANSWERS HAVE BEEN AROUND FOR A LONG TIME

I believe your attitude is your choice
I believe you can choose out of major disease
I believe your mental state can be healthy
& I believe
YOU CAN ALTER YOUR DNA

DIANNE HOFFMANN
I am here to make your tomorrow better than today

Reports by Researcher
R. NEIL VOSS

Affirmations included

No One Thing™
By Dianne Hoffmann

For further information contact the author at:

No One Thing
c/o Hoffmann Publishing
1296 Oak Hill Circle
Provo, Utah 84604
e-mail: no_one_thing@comcast.net

Book Design by John Morris-Reihl www.artntech.com

PRINTER and DISTRIBUTOR in The United States of America by
Lightning Source Inc. (US)
1246 Heil Quaker Blvd.
La Vergne, TN USA 37086
615) 213-5815

Dianne Hoffmann
NO ONE THING to master your life

1. Author 2. Title
Library of Congress Catalog Card Number:
ISBN: 978-0-0-9795246-1-5

GRATITUDE GOES TO

Susan Bliss	Theda Therapist: right brain utilization
Gale & Bob Stringham	Psychotherapist and Counselor
Judi Moore	Good friend: integrative doctor
Dian Voss	Good friend: advisor
Chance, Cologne	My Children have taught me
Chase, Chi & Charney	Unconditional love, determination, non-judgmental, tenderness, gratitude, faith.
Canyon	Guardian Angel, 4-13-85 to 12-8-01
Tiger	Soul Mate: My Love, My Husband, My Friend
Impact Training	taught me to be in my excellence.
Synapse Experience	gave me a taste of success.
Experience	Life taught me wisdom.
Baby Girl in my Dream	(born to another), taught me to release and let go.
Carma	This past, I must remember. The present I cherish. That way I can pay it forward.
Mae Dvorak	Computer consultant
Dora Fay Hill Sorenson	My Mother loved so much (Angel)
Doyle ReVo Sorenson	My Father. I now understand him
Siblings	Julia-Mae-Carolyn-Carma-Antone-Alayna-Nathan-Sunshine
Siblings in heaven (angels)	Doyle-Darrel-Anthony-Owen-Kenneth

I am grateful for people I meet. Most have shown me a mirror of myself, even when I didn't care to look, and others have given me wings. Thank You

To Elaine my New Friend So glad I met you. Deanne Hoffmann

iii

TABLE OF CONTENTS

A Thought I like to live by

A NEW DAY

This is the beginning of a new day.

God has given me this day to use as I will.

I can waste it or use it for good,

But what I do today is important,

Because I am exchanging a day of my life for it.

When tomorrow comes, this day will be gone forever;

Leaving in its place something I have traded for it.

I want it to be gain and not loss,

Good, and not evil; success, and not failure,

In order that I shall not regret the price that

I have paid for it.

Forward

The purpose of this book is not to give you detailed information about the ways of healing physical or mental conditions. The body itself has the power to heal itself. The things we do, to and for our body, assist in that process. There is much information in books from people who have researched many avenues of assisting the body. Most of us with a mental capacity over seven know that we need air containing oxygen and water to live. We are also aware that we need to intake food and expel waste. Most of us know that we need touch and interaction. In the scheme of things, there are a number of categories that promote health: physical, mental, emotional and spiritual (our inner knowing), and we learn by feeling (kinesthetic), hearing (auditory), and seeing (visual). All the ways of learning will be in this book and we will be covering healing in the above categories.

What about the water we drink, the air we breathe, the food we eat and the daily interaction? Most of us can live in good health by integrating the things we know into our lives.

What some people do not know is the necessity for *clean* air, *pure* water, foods that supply all the *necessary nutrients* that keep our body healthy.

Because most of the earth has been depleted of minerals, the food we are eating is deficient. It may look like a fruit, vegetable or nut but the same vital nutrients are not in the same concentration as they were thousands of years ago when man lived to be close to 1000 years.

One purpose of this book is to give you healthful hints and healing modalities that can assist your body in being healthy and happy, which in turn, contributes to better peace and harmony.

Another purpose of writing this book is to organize my thoughts as an author and to make sense of the life-experience that I and others have endured. The first 2 decades of my life were quite traumatic and deep seated injuries were alleviated by writing about them. There is a healing process that occurs as one organizes and re-views the occurrences and begins to understand.

My experiences have taught me much in the way of health on a mental and physical note. There will be no blame---only the way it is. The first remembrance of dis-ease in my body was not being able to breathe through my nose, nausea and severe ear aches. My parents taped my mouth shut to force me to breathe through my nose. For survival's sake, I learned to sneak really well. I moistened the tape with my tongue. I could only get occasional sips of air. I learned to hold my breath for long periods of time. Was I feeling that my parents didn't care? That they thought I was a liar? That I need to sneak to survive? And could I really trust them? I could trust the priesthood because a priesthood blessing is what stopped my earaches at the age of eleven or twelve. I had to figure things out by myself.

Because of what I had experienced and because of the way I perceived things, I had become a semi-invalid by the age of 29. I was up 4 hours a day and down for 20. Most of the 20 hours was spent sleeping. My skin coloring was turning green. I was septic. Most of my normal body functions were not working. I had to concentrate on all the involuntary functions. I woke up in the middle of the night gasping for air. I did not breathe without effort. I was not eliminating. Getting up out of bed caused my heart to race and beat so loudly I could not only feel it but thought I was hearing it as well. I was depressed. I cried a lot. An M.D. prescribed Valium. I tore up the prescription. I wanted to get well. Not cover it up. One day I said, "Lord, please take me or make me well." I said it with total conviction. I was septic and my skin was turning green in color. I was introduced to herbs and a friend suggested I go on a cleanse (fast). So many toxins were released into my blood stream that I almost checked out of life. I fought and won. I had chiropractic and acupressure. I read, studied and put my research into use. My involuntary functions began to improve. I started to eat and not worry about being fat. I gained muscle and did *not* get rid of any fat, so I had weight gain. My exercise existed of lifting my legs and arms in bed, getting up and down as needed with a mental attitude that my body was responding in some way. I refused to over-exercise no matter what the outside pressure, but I did not give up. As I studied, I learned of many therapies that were very beneficial. I learned that there are at least 3 main categories of herbs: medicinal, food (non addicting), and poisonous. I'm not going into that except to say that a reputable herbal company is not going to package poisonous herbs and there are a lot of good companies out there.

In the following pages are the beneficial therapies that I have experienced.

Prologue

Most of the pioneers in health have had major health issues that were not being solved by doctors. There was research done and much testing. Discoveries were made by these pioneers long before the medical profession started paying any attention. Once a discovery has been made, the FDA requires years and years of testing. Even then some medications have been recalled due to failure. A pharmacist will stand by the product he dispenses saying that medication is derived from the same plant as the alternative ways of healing. But there is a difference. The pharmaceuticals take the active ingredient out of the plant and prepare it in easy to use tablets. The problem is that without the rest of the plants' inert ingredient, that supports the active ingredients, there may be many side effects from prescription drugs. Pharmaceuticals also use synthetically duplicate active ingredients, which could also be another detriment to us since the molecules in synthetics spin to the left. Left spin is life depleting and right spin is live enhancing. The value of each will be discussed later in the book.

There are benefits of both alternative modes of healing and standard care where there is tight control by the AMA which regulates what Doctors can prescribe. Doctors generally diagnose and dispense medicine in times of great need. There is a need for that.

Physical, mental, emotional and spiritual are often entwined in that they all influence each other. On a daily basis I make creative choices that help to increase my health and I am sure, cuts expense on medical care and saves me so much time and money. Sometimes we get busy and do not listen to our body and wait until we are forced to use emergency means that do not always bring us to total health. There are many ways to create and maintain good health that do not require a lot of time or money: possibly no more than you are spending right now. The products and devices that I use, I use to bring me good health and sustain the health that I have. I will show you how to increase your physical, mental, emotional and spiritual selves by introducing you to some fun and rewarding therapies and activities.

Preface

I appreciate my life-experience that created who I am today. I have been through countless deficiencies in physical, mental, emotional and spiritual areas. As many pioneers in the health field, I have done intensive research and learned from other peoples' trial and error. I have been blessed with a type of wisdom that causes me to dedicate myself to assist people in being both physically and mentally healthy. I think of the song by a group of well known singers. "'Heal the World' make it a better place...... This is my focus. I have withstood the winds of time. There are still winds blowing me in directions that I am uncomfortable with, but I will prevail.

There will be a lot of things in this book that you already know. If it inspires you do the things you already know, that is good enough.

There are things you may not agree with. That's O.K. too. Nothing in this book will harm you and some or most of it may be of great assistance.

I am also aware that if you reject what is being said in this book, there is a good reason for it. Life's experiences assist people to grow. If you need an experience to grow or to assist others in growing, you may subconsciously want to remain ill and you may either reject it or it won't work on you anyway. It is for you to choose. If you decide to be ill, celebrate. You made a conscious choice. Be grateful or make a new choice and be grateful for that one.

Books have been written on each of the therapies, activities, devices and products, ideas and many more. There is no reason to duplicate these authors. I would never take away from their research.

This book is only an introduction to the many things that we have available to us. I've made an effort to learn everything I can; and if it makes perfect sense, I have usually tried it. I have my own personal favorites and you may find your own personal favorites among the pages that follow.

NO ONE THING
To master your life

SECTION ONE

CHAPTER ONE

LET'S TAKE A LOOK AT THE HEALTH INDUSTRY

When we are seeking for a resolution to a problem, there are decisions to be made. There are some options that people choose for health. There is no one thing that will secure optimum health. What you eat and when you eat is as important as the people you seek after to assist you in retaining or regaining your health.

There are people that think that an allergy causes sneezing, itchy eyes, rashes, drowsiness and such. They do. And Anti-allergy medications can alleviate these symptoms, yet cause drowsiness. There are actually over 100 different allergic reactions to allergens. A contributing factor is often a saturation of the thing that you are allergic to and allergens are frequently passed on to offspring. Some allergic reactions are: feeling tired, passing gas, addictions, joint pain, head aches, burning eyes, nasal clogs, ear aches, body odor and bad breath, to name a few. The rotation diet can lessen allergic reactions tremendously.

Medical Doctors: With years of study and practice a doctor can compare your symptoms with other patients' and can usually come up with a pretty good diagnosis. Because of this the doctor can also narrow down what may help you with regard to medication. There is a risk of side effects that medication can cause (depending on the doctor) but there is great skill in the art of surgery. His practice is bound by the AMA and the FDA and he has little ability to stretch out and do something more.

Dr. Lars-Erik Essen, a dermatologist in Halsinborg, Sweden, pioneered the use of bee products for skin conditions. He treated many of his patients successfully for acne. Dr. Essen says, "Through transcutaneous nutrition, bee pollen exerts a profound biological effect. It seems to prevent premature aging of the cells and stimulates growth of new skin tissue. It offers effective protection against dehydration and injects new life into dry cells. It smoothes away wrinkles and stimulates a life-giving blood supply to all skin cells."

1

Dr. Essen, a leading authority on skin speaks out about his profession.

Here is a case of medicinal value by Dr. Essen:

"A doctor is treating a case of infectious disease by the conventional methods. The determining factor for a successful result of this kind of treatment is to identify the kind of bacteria considered responsible for the infection in question. When the intruder is identified, the patient is given a specific chemical or antibiotic drug, which, as a rule, accomplishes the immediate results: the bacteria are destroyed and the patient is free from the symptoms.

After a while, it may happen that the same patient will turn up with a new infection. The diagnosis shows that either it is a question of the same kind of bacteria, which, at this time, however, is already immune to the specific drug, or there are new bacteria involved. Accordingly, new and more potent drugs are prescribed, which bring about immediate results, as far as the fighting bacteria is concerned. But in spite of the "success" of the treatment, the patient's resistance to infection seems to progressively weaken and various complications set in. Now, perhaps, such potent drugs as cortisone-pain-killer and symptom-remover-and other highly toxic synthetic drugs enter the picture The body, already weakened by the disease, must now, in addition, cope with the toxic and damaging side effects of the poisonous drugs.

Then, one day, we stand by the deathbed surprised and shocked. The patient had received all the correct treatments in accordance with medical science's conventional practices and regulations. The laboratory tests prove that we made no errors? Bacteria samples showed that the bacteria, which our treatment was aimed at, were 'successfully' eradicated. As far as the direct cause of the symptoms was concerned (the bacteria) our treatment was a complete success. The only problem was that the patient died? We succeeded in killing the bacteria, but we failed to save the host organism, where our war on bacteria was so successful. It also could be said that the treatment was successful, but unfortunately, as a result of the treatment and resultant complications, the patient died. Or, 'The operation was successful, but the patient didn't survive.'

Now, actually, this kind of a result is not so surprising, is it? After all, what did we treat? Our treatment was directed at micro-organisms which we considered pathogenic or disease-causing. In the meantime, the biological environment for this micro-organism, the host organism, the living, delicate, sensitive, and easily damaged human body has actually been completely neglected. The man hardly comes into the picture at all. What we actually treat today are diseases, not diseased people. The sick body, however, is subject to very different biological laws than those which could be applied in primitive germ war with chemical and antibiotic germ-killers.

A parallel to this can be seen in today's damage and destruction of life and natural environments as a result of man's indiscriminate use of insecticides and other poisonous chemicals. Is there any intelligent human being who is so naïve as to assume that these poisons will be less devastating to the human body, with its endlessly more intricate and delicate living mechanism? The biological laws of life are quite different from the laws which regulate chemical reactions observed in laboratory tubes. When we fail to see the difference between the two, catastrophic conditions will be the result, and we have to accept the consequences of our unwise actions."

I am not suggesting that there is no value in medicine. I am suggesting that when we do need to see a medical practitioner, we also need to build the body and choose good healing techniques to rebuild after the medical treatments. We can also do things that *keep* us healthy and avoid getting sick.

We have talked about traditional medicine as directed by most medical doctors. Some doctors have the philosophy of "Biological Medicine." It is comforting to know that there are medical doctors who use this approach. Dr. Essen continues:

"When the biologically oriented physician is confronted with a case of infectious disease his approach and his actions are entirely different. For him, bacteria and viruses which are present in certain infections, are phenomena of secondary interest. He considers them only as symptomatic factors in relation to the host organism (the patient) and his body as a biological environment. All his attention is directed towards the patient. His primary aim is to employ every measure available to increase the power of resistance within the host organism and avoid causing it any damage. The first principle of the art of healing, enunciated already by the Father of Medicine, Hippocrates, 'Primum est nil nocere'-the most important thing of all is that treatment must do no harm-is violated in present-day medical practice more than in any other period of medical history.

The biologically oriented doctor is aware that with chemical and antibiotic drugs he will always cause damage to the host organism's biological milieu, even though with such treatments he can achieve a temporary effect. Therefore, he avoids to the utmost the use of such drugs in the management of simple and harmless infections. To treat a common cold or a sore throat with, for example, penicillin, for him is a crime against the fundamental rules of health. Instead, his attention is directed to increasing the body's own resistance with all the natural, harmless, biological methods of treatment which are available."

Biological Medicine has been in existence over 20 years with an excellent record. The doctor will encourage the patient and give him/her proper aid in the form of rest, fasting, wholesome diet, and other biological measures, which strengthen the patients own healing power to win the battle. Biological treatments raise the general resistance of patients and as a rule they will become more immune to infections in the future. If you know of a good doctor that practices Biological Medicine in your area, let me know and I will pass it along to my readers.

Holistic guides: There are a great number of publications and literature that can assist a person in choosing for themselves what foods and herbs to use to assist the body in healing itself.

Nothing can heal your body but your body and your intentions. There are less side effects with natural foods and herbs than with medications. There are many people who wish to combine a medical doctor's expertise with the natural way mentioned above.

Homeopathic remedies have been very successful in assisting the body to heal itself. Many people are turning to homeopathic remedies when a doctor has given up on them or when they have done everything medically possible. They cost less and have little or no side effects. Many professional institutes have caught on, and are taking a holistic approach to treatment. I have had much success with homeopathy. I do not know if The Nevada Clinic of Preventive Medicine in Las Vegas where I received care still exists; however, there are reputable places available.

Acupuncture has been used for thousands of years in China and practitioners in the US have also found it to be extremely effective. China uses it for preventive well being. Doctors in China get paid only for their people who are well and can work. The doctor reads the patients' pulse with his fingers to determine if any of the 12 meridians are out of balance. This way the doctor knows which organs of the body, if any, are headed for disease.

There are ways to get in balance without acupuncture if you are still in relatively good condition. Certain exercises, movements and tapping can assist. More of that will be discussed later.

SECTION ONE
CHAPTER TWO
THERAPIES

Sometimes there are reasons for alternating techniques and therapies. Some of these are boredom, diminishing benefit over long term use, becoming allergic (over 100 symptoms), lack of convenience, cost, time restraints, difficulty etc.

Many therapies are simply the use of energy and intention with heart and mind. The mind is used to gather information and the heart is used for processing information. Simply put.

Some of the therapies for Mental and Physical issues are:

Affirmation Therapy: It has been said that for every negative you say or hear, it takes seven positives to cancel the negative. It has also been said that affirmations sometimes are best heard subliminally. Some people argue with them. When you are ready to read affirmations, read them over and over again. You will find it helpful as you begin to believe them. You can use the ones at the end of this book or create your own affirmations by using the ones at the end of this book as a guide. Use no negatives when creating your own. It weakens the effectiveness of the affirmation. Think of it this way. If I tell you to not think of an elephant, what is the first thing you think of? A young child and your subconscious do not hear negatives. They will close the door if you tell them *"Don't close the door."* Don't is a negative and they do not hear it. Example: Leave the door open. I am thin. I am healthy.

A Story to Tell

John was close to death. He had no will to live and was barely breathing. He was so stiff; he looked dead. We placed a tape recorder at his bedside and played subliminal affirmations with peaceful, life-giving music over and over throughout the night. John survived the night and the music and subliminal affirmations kept playing throughout the day and night for several days. He recovered.

6

Aroma Therapy: Essential Oils are generally used for aromatherapy. It is a bit easier than building a terrarium and planting all manner of marvelous herbs and flowers. The essential oils should be of highest quality and 100% pure and natural. The best oils come from wild or organic plants.

Essential oils are used for healing the physical body by restoring energy balance and have a strong subconscious effect on emotions. They are comforting, elevating and soothing to the spirit.

No more than 5 drops of the essential oils are recommended on the skin. The ones that can go on the skin without being diluted are: Birch, chamomile, carrot, cedar wood, cistus, clary sage, eucalyptus, geranium, lavender, lemon, lime, marjoram, myrtle, neroli, orange, palmarosa, petitgrain, rosemary, rosewood, sandalwood, tangerine, vetiver and ylang ylang. Blending oils are more efficient if you blend with similar or complementary oils. Here are a few Essential Oils and what they have been historically used for:

Plant	Physical healing	Emotional feeling
Basil	Digestive system and intestinal infections	Brain stimulant, mental fatigue, depression, mental strain
Bergamot	Digestive, antispasmodic	Uplifting, lightening, depression, anxiety
Birch	Kidneys, joints, analgesic, diuretic, depurative, rheumatism, arthritis	
Chamomile	Female affections, anti-inflammatory, calming	Depression, irritability, insomnia, hysteria, hypersensitivity
Cedarwood	Respiratory system, (eczema)	Anxiety, nervous tension
Clary	Female genitals, menstruations, frigidity, lucorrhea	Relaxant, euphoric, stress, tension, aphrodisiac

Clove	antiseptic, dyspepsia, gastric fermentation, wounds,	Poor memory, intellectual, asthenia, impotence
Cypress	Astringent, diuretic, varicose, asthma, whooping cough	
Eucalyptus	Respiratory system, expectorant, antiseptic, deodorizer	Invigorating, balancing
Fir	Respiratory, antiseptic, expectorant, vulnerary	Appeasing, fortifying
Geranium	Kidney, antidiabetic, stimulant of adrenal cortex, astringent	Uplifting, anxiety, nervous tension, depression
Juniper	Detoxifying, diuretic toxin & fluid, retention/cellulite, rheumatism, urinary infections	Nervous tonic, poor memory, nervous fatigue, cleansing
Lavender	The universal oil: calming, antiseptic, healing	Soothing, appeasing, energy balance
Lemon	Stimulant, tonic, controls secretions, stomach, blood fluid	Refreshing, optimistic, fearless, strengthening
Marjoram	Antispasmodic, calming, sedative, digestive, asthma, bronchitis	Insomnia, grief, neurasthenia, nervous tension, anxiety, migraine
Myrrh		Comforting, fortifying, elevating, charkas, aged skin)
Orange	Digestive, sedative, indigestion	Appeasing, oversensitivity, nervous tension
Palmarosa	Antiseptic, imbalance calming, physiological skin, hydrating, wrinkles	uplifting

8

Patchouli	Cell regenerator, eczema, impetigo, dermatitis, wrinkles, fungicidal, dandruff	Depression, anxiety
Peppermint	Digestive system, liver intestines, nausea, vomiting, cold cough, fainting, (cleansing, decongesting)	Brain stimulant, headache, migraine, mental fatigue
Petitgrain	Painful digestion	Nervous sedative, intellectual, stimulant, poor memory
Pine	Respiratory system, pectoral, hepatic & urinary, antiseptic	Warming, reviving, comforting, emotional stress
Rosemary	Liver, gall-bladder, cardio-tonic, dry skin, rejuvenating, dandruff, hair loss	Mental fatigue, mental strain, poor memory, sadness
Rosewood	Calming, emollient, cellular stimulant, wrinkles, scars, pimples	Soothing, euphoric
Sage	Liver, gall-bladder, wrinkles, eczema, females genitals,	Nervous tonic, low energy, neurasthenia, vertigo
Sandalwood	Male genitals, genitor-urinary, affections	Aphrodisiac, deep relaxant, stimulant of psychic centers
Tea Tree	Fungicidal, anti-virus, anti-infections, immune stimulant, fungus/candida	
Thyme	General stimulant, infections & pulmonary diseases, rheumatism, arthritis, cold, flu	Brain stimulant, neurasthenia, depression, fatigue
Ylang-Ylang	Hypo tensor	Aphrodisiac, euphoric, anger, frustration, insomnia

There are other Aromatherapy charts and books for additional information.

Breathing Patterns Therapy: I learned the breathing method from Tom who is a Martial Arts Black Belt and instructor for the State of Utah Self-Defense Training. In all breathing methods it is important to breathe in as deeply as you can and blow out as deeply as you can. Do not be concerned as to how deeply you breathe. The depth will increase. If you are used to breathing shallow or holding your breath a lot, you may tend to cough. Cough and keep going. Here is the pattern:

As you inhale, count 1, 2, 3, 4, 5, 6, 7 ,8. Hold for 1, 2, 3, 4. Exhale 1, 2, 3,4, 5, 6, 7, 8. Hold for 1, 2, 3, 4. Start over. If you can not do 8 inhale 4 hold 8 exhale 4 hold, start with 4-2-4-2 or 6-3-6-3. What ever you can do is well enough. Keep practicing and your endurance in many things will increase. If you need a nap and do not have time for one, or if you are expecting a stressful encounter or situation, try the above exercise.

Chakra Therapy: If the Chakras are open and balanced, the positive qualities will display themselves. If the Chakras are out of balance or blocked the negative qualities will display themselves. Following are the 7 Chakras with their locations, colors for strengthening, functions, positive qualities and negative qualities. You can use the colors corresponding to your birthday or use these general colors for the charkas.

1.   Base or root Chakra: Base of the spine (coccyx)
       Color is Red.   Black is secondary
       Gives vitality to the physical body, life force, survival, self preservation, instincts
       Qualities: Success, mastery of the body, stability, health, courage, patience
       Negative: Self-centeredness, insecurity, violence, greed, anger, tension in spine, constipation

2.	Navel or Sacral plexus Chakra: Lower abdomen to navel
	Color is Orange
	Procreation, assimilation of food, physical force and vitality, sexuality
	Qualities: emotions, desire, pleasure, change, movement, new ideas, family, working harmoniously and creatively with others
	Negative: over-indulgence in food or sex, confusion, purposelessness, jealousy, impotence

3.	Solar Plexus Chakra:	Above navel,	below the chest
	Color is Yellow
	Vitalize the sympathetic nervous system, digestive processes, metabolism, emotions
	Qualities: personal power, authority, energy, mastery of desire, self control, radiance, humor, laughter, immortality
	Negative: anger, fear, hate, digestive problems, too much emphasis on power or recognition

4.	Heart Chakra:	Center of chest
	Color is Green.	Pink is secondary
	Energizes the blood and physical body and life force of the higher self
	Qualities: unconditional love, forgiveness, compassion, understanding, balance, acceptance, peace, openness, harmony, contentment
	Negative: represses love, emotionally unstable, heart problems

5.	Throat Chakra	Throat area
	Color is Sky Blue
	Speech, sound, vibrations, communication
	Qualities: true communication, creative expression in speech, writing, integration, peace, truth, wisdom, loyalty, honesty, reliability, gentleness, kindness
	Negative: knowledge used unwisely, ignorance, lack of discernment, depression, thyroid problems

6.   Brow Chakra: Third Eye   Center of forehead
Color is Indigo (Dark Blue)
Vitalizes the Cerebellum (lower brain) and central nervous system, vision
Qualities: intuition, insight, imagination, peace of mind, wisdom, devotion, soul realization
Negatives: lack of concentration, fear, cynicism, tension, headaches, eye problems, bad dreams

7.   Crown Chakra: Top of head
Color is Violet
Vitalizes the Cerebrum (upper brain)
Qualities: idealism, selfless service, spiritual will, inspiration, unity, divinity, wisdom, inspiration
Negative: lack of inspiration, confusion, depression, alienation, hesitation to serve, senility

The Chakras can be opened and balanced through meditation, energy work and Layers of Light products.

Colon Therapy: Because of the way most people eat, the body does not completely discard all the matter in the colon. In fact, if we do not keep the colon cleaned out, the intestines often fail to function properly. Many clients of colonic therapists have reported more energy, clearer skin and eyes, increased elimination through the kidney, skin and bowel, relief from gas, and a toned and better working bowel. This makes perfect sense.

How long can a fruit, vegetable, meat, or milk stay on the kitchen counter before it putrefies at room temperature. When you put the same things in your body, it is 98.6 f. Did you know that your intestines are actually porous? Often when a person gets a headache, it is caused by poisons excreting from the intestinal walls.

Color Therapy: Simple to do. It assists with dream therapy, rainbow therapy and can also bring out your ability to visualize. Get out the crayons and paper and start with a rainbow. Draw an arch for a guide and start coloring the arches, making a rainbow with the colors of your choice. You may want to advance to water colors and acrylics or even take an art class. It will heighten your abilities. If

12

you practice enough, you should be able to visualize with your eyes closed.

Laboratory tests prove that each color has its' own vibration and benefits. This vibratory energy in color affects your health, comfort, happiness and safety.

Color, in the form of light is part of the electro-magnetic spectrum. Lights can supply energy to the body. Light color therapy can restore health, energy and good nutrition. Light therapy will be covered later. Whether you use colored lights, crayons and/or other color mediums, you will receive great benefits. The following colors and representations are here for you to consider.

Colors to Play with

Red: Courage/Life. Red is the color of exciting energy and of accepting and giving. It is an action color with motion to get things done and is especially good to follow Royal Blue, the leadership color.

Orange: Wisdom/Decision-making. This color adds warmth and combines colors of red and yellow and helps a body normalize. Increases energy and represents thoughtfulness and consideration.

Green: Abundance/Agape Love. Green is the healing color of grass and represents a desire to have profound healing: physically and mentally. It works for the sympathetic nervous System and increases vitality, represents abundance in nature, helps with general healing, restoration and balance. It is the master healer. Agape Love is also healing.

Pink: Love/Relationship. It is the color of giving your loving thoughts and actions. It affects the mind more than the body and encourages joy, comfort and companionship. It is the key to abundance.

Purple: Peace/Healing. It desires enlightenment of the higher laws of the universe. Spiritual powers increase. It is useful in purifying the body and helping maintain potassium-sodium balance.

Light Blue: Spirituality. It is the color of the heavens and shows desire to communicate with the universe and with God, which brings serenity. It represents inspiration and healing love, which is soothing. Your pulse lowers and exhaling deepens, giving a feeling of release and retreat. It is an emotional sedative color.

Royal Blue: Leadership. This color is for ordained leadership callings to accomplish special missions or callings in life, including those who feel duty to a higher source and those who may be rebellious in accepting their chosen path.

Yellow: Fun/Spirituality. Yellow is bright, optimistic, cheerful and friendly. This color represents a merry sunshine soul who wants to give happiness and enjoy life and is often tired of the serious side of life. They want to "Let go and let God" with faith.

White: Ultimate Purity. Brilliance of light is connected to the Savior. Also used for emotional release.

Black: Controls emotions/Calms. It is the absence of all color, and has the lowest vibration of all colors. Color for funeral

Brown: Stability/Focus: This is a grounding color. This is the color people select when they want stability and want to be on solid ground. It represents integration, offering and even sacrifice.

Gold: Power: It is a powerful empowering color. Added to green, Gold has a profound healing effect and makes a big impact.

Aqua: Peace/Tranquility. This color is for those who want peace and tranquility. It also assists those who want to resolve all conflict and discord out of their life and have only the smooth vibrations of calmness. It is both relaxing and calming.

There is no need to use white in your rainbow if you are using a white back ground but make sure you use all of the above colors. You can add to them.

Some of the colors for Feng-shui are a little different. We'll cover that a little later.

Dream Therapy: Drink plenty of pure water when you go to sleep and drink it when you awake. Have writing material with you and jot down what you remember each time you awake.

Before you fall asleep, think of what you want to dream about. Start the story line and keep it going through the first stages of sleep. You can control your dream in these stages, and when REM comes along you will not necessarily be in control at first, but keep it up and you will be able to create what you desire in a more effective and effortless way. Your dreams can actually create new memories to crowd out the old.

Exercise Therapy: Increases oxygenation and endorphins. There are many fun activities that you can do that will work. Some of those are: Bouncing on a Trampoline, Jumping rope, Walking, Swimming and all of those favorites that you have always wanted to experience.

A Story to Tell

As a soft drop-shot came over the net, Louis raced in for the return. He extended his racket to scoop up the ball and felt a burning knifelike pain suddenly shoot into both his calves. It spread up to his thighs and his legs went numb.

A month earlier on his wedding anniversary, he and his wife were celebrating in the Virgin Islands. On that happy day, he swam two miles and was on the court for another two hours. At 72 years old he was still competing in tennis against people 30 years younger.

After numerous tests, the prognosis was occlusions of the femoral arteries on both legs caused by a buildup of plaque that extended all the way up to the aorta.

Louis' diseased arteries could be operated on, but it would be very expensive and very dangerous. If the surgery did not work, gangrene could set in and he could lose both legs.

The doctor paused and said "You know, you're in pretty good shape for your age. I want people like you to work me out of my job. If you'll walk at least a mile every day, I think your body will cure the clogged-artery problem by itself."

Louis decided to try it but after seven months Louis became really depressed. The weather was bitterly cold and every step seemed harder. Louis called the doctor and told him that he was considering the operation. An appointment was made and the doctor kept Louis waiting nearly two hours. As Louis waited, a parade of people passed by him: some missing legs, some in wheelchairs, others struggling to stand up. When Louis finally got to see the doctor, he told the doctor his waiting room looked like a Civil War emergency room. "That was exactly what I wanted you to see," the doctor said. "Now get back to walking." Louis did.

Louis and his wife moved to Florida where the weather was warm until mid-June when the weather in N.Y. became sunny and warm. He changed his diet to avoid red meat, cut back on fatty foods and sodium and ate more fruits and vegetables for breakfast, lunch and dinner.

Although it will be necessary for Louis to continue his activity to keep the disease from recurring, he really enjoys his new way of life. He encourages others to ask their doctor if they too could avoid invasive surgery by doing something as simple as walking. The healing powers of our bodies are there, just waiting to be used.

Hydro-Therapy: Hydro means water. A whole house water system is a plus for every home. There are three water therapies: drinking, soaking, and colonic. Tap water is not usually used for therapies except in soaking because of the ingredients added to the water for

16

cleansing or detoxing. If you use plastic for drinking, it is best to use a high density plastic or grade 7 of the low density plastics.

1. Drinking. The body is made up of 75% water. Since we excrete it, we need to replace it. Your body needs water whether you are thirsty or not. In fact, if you get thirsty, you have waited too long. Among the professionals who suggest the use of water are: Doctors, Massage Therapists, Chiropractors and Herbalists. Most health professionals do. Many people believe that the body can utilize water best by drinking small amounts of water often. Water is the transport mechanism for oxygen, hydrogen, minerals and enzymes. If you drink more than you can utilize it ends up in the bladder. If you drink 4 ounces every half hour and you are up for 10 hours a day, you got it. Make a habit and it is simple. Just keep on sipping away. You may be pleasantly surprised at how much better you feel.

Sometimes the body needs to flush toxins and unwanted waste. You may also be more physically active. In this case, more water is good.

2. Skin: Water with vinegar, bleach, or salt added to the bath is a means where-by the toxins can be cleansed from the skin. It is also absorbed by the skin and provides you with a deep cleanse.

3. Colon: This was covered in Colon Therapy. However, the colon is so important to have cleaned out that it will not hurt to repeat it in part. Sometimes the body doesn't discard all the matter in the intestines with the way we eat. In fact if we do not keep the colon cleaned out, the intestines can often fail to function properly. Many clients of colonic therapists have reported more energy, clearer skin and eyes, increased elimination through the kidneys, skin and bowel, relief from gas, and a toned and better working bowel. It makes sense.

The intestines are where the immune system does 80% of its' work, so if your colon is functioning at less efficiency than desired, how is your body going to fight off un-invited guests.

Hypnotherapy and age regression: These therapies have proven to be of great value when working with the mind. Every human being has faced many traumas in life that cause them to make certain decisions at the time of the trauma.

A one year old child who was beaten fiercely by her father made a decision at that time that she would do whatever it takes to keep that from happening again. She used sex to get what she wanted. She lied, cheated, robbed and used men and degraded the men in her life.

Children in abuse make decisions at the time of the abuse to avoid or get even to lessen the pain. Often, they do not know why they do things. They are simply compelled.

When I went through hypnotherapy and age regression, I was able to change all of the concepts of who I was and became who I wanted to be. All my thinking patterns changed by creating a new memory. All my growing up years were painful. When I went through age regression I mentally went through each of my early years and wrote a whole new story with imagery.

Every child makes decisions when they are young. The only thing they can cognitively do at that young age is decide to make the pain stop. Their decision making skills have not been developed fully and whatever those decisions are, affects their whole life. They usually do not know why they do the things they do throughout their life. They just feel the compelling need to do it. With hypnotherapy, age regression and Rapid Eye Therapy, lives are dramatically changed. Beliefs are altered. Freedom is attained. This therapy can be categorized in all modes of health: Physical, mental and spiritual. It is so important for those who have been through major trauma to seek out modes of healing to eliminate harmful behavior. Sometimes we block off the trauma because the memory of it is too painful. Often the memory does not have to come back for you to heal. Often, it does.

Laughter Therapy: The saying "Laughter is the best medicine" is right on. A man had cancer and was given 6 months to live. He thought "chuck this" and he did. He quit his job, stayed home and watched funny movies pretty much non stop. He laughed so hard that the cancer actually subsided. Laughter is healing: Physically and Mentally. It helps to bring in more oxygen. It's fun and very cost effective. Lighten up you serious souls. You'll be healthier for it. Just for fun, I'm going to give you a little humor. It may not make you laugh but it is light hearted and might make you feel the need to go find something to make you laugh.

- An Amish boy and his father were visiting a shopping mall for the first time. They were amazed by almost everything they saw, but especially by two shiny, silver walls that could move apart and back together again.

  The boy asked his father, "What is this, father?"

  The father (never having seen an elevator before) responded, "Son, I have never seen anything like this in my life, I don't know what it is."

  While the boy and his father were watching wide-eyed, an old lady in a wheel chair rolled up to the moving walls and pressed a button. The walls opened and the lady rolled between them into a small room. The walls closed and the boy and his father watched small circles of lights with numbers above the walls light up. They continued to watch the circles light up in the reverse direction. The walls opened up again and a beautiful 24 year old woman stepped out.

  The father moved his black hat back on his head, then said to his son. "Go get your mother."

- The following is a courtroom exchange between a defense attorney and a farmer with a bodily injury claim.

Attorney "At the scene of the accident, did you tell the constable you had never felt better in your life?"

Farmer: That's right"
Attorney: "Well, then, how is it that you are now claiming you were seriously injured when my client's auto hit your wagon?"

Farmer: When the constable arrived, he went over to my horse, who had a broken leg, and shot him. Then he went over to Rover, my dog, who was all banged up, and shot him. When he asked me how I felt, I just thought under the circumstances, it was a wise choice of words to say "I've never felt better in my life."

- Two extremely old ladies were sitting in rocking chairs and one said to the other, "I'm getting so old that all my friends in heaven will think I didn't make it."

- "When I die I'd like to go peacefully in my sleep…like my grandfather, not screaming…like the passengers in his car."

- A mother was teaching her 3 year old daughter The Lords Prayer. For several evenings at bedtime she repeated it after her mother. One night the little girl said she wanted to do it solo. The mother listened with pride as she carefully enunciated each word right up to the end "Lead us not into temptation" she prayed "but deliver us some E-mail.

Light Therapy: Just a little on this. Check into it if you are interested. There are actually two therapies called light therapy and they are totally different. One is with actual fixture lighting. The yellow lighting as in fluorescent lighting is very draining on the energy. Some put a magnet next to it to taper down the effect. Some choose to get full spectrum lighting. Some fluorescents eliminate the yellow and are better. The sun's light is the best for health except even that has damaging rays to the skin.

The other Light Therapy is referring to emotional lighting such as in "Breathe in light and breathe out darkness." People use this in mental healing. This is sometimes referred to as Christ-Light. Love and light are synonymous with this type of healing.

Magnetic Therapy: It is reported that thousands of years ago people lived nearly 1000 years. Today we have medical technology that can assist us in living to nearly 100 years. Even then the quality of life is not there. Scientific studies show that there is a correlation between the length of life and the magnetic field.

The magnetism of the earth has been declining and the length of quality of life has been declining as well. Have you ever noticed that babies and pets love the outdoors?

There are positive and negative ions in magnetism. The positive ions create high energy and the negative ions create restfulness. When it is balanced, it creates a healthy state.

Our homes and offices have so many positive ions that the magnetism is completely off balance. Positive ions manifest themselves in electricity. Everything around us is electric unless we go outdoors.

One very effective way to keep the magnetic field in balance is to sleep on a magnetic pad. Another benefit of magnetic therapy is that the blood pumps through the veins and capillaries at a higher rate causing better oxygenation and causing the nutrients to be delivered to the cells in a more timely manner.

Nikken is a company that offers many magnetic devices and products that assist in keeping the blood flowing and oxygenated. Oxygen does not get to all parts of the body in some cases. Diabetics often become amputees due to poor circulation (of oxygen).

The products that Nikken has to offer are beautiful jewelry, socks, shoes, thermal underwear, sleep pads, sleep comforter, air purifier, water purifier, back massager, devices for feet, wrists, knees, feet, eyes, head and face.

Some people would rather go through procedures that are paid for by insurance even though it does not make them feel better, look better or act better. Sometimes it is a matter of money.

Massage Therapy: There are a number of styles of massage. Pick the one you like and go for it or rotate. I have had a number of different styles. Go for the one you are in the mood for at the time. You will most probably feel pampered, uplifted and at peace. With massage, you get 2 therapies. I do not know a good massage therapist that doesn't have good music.

A few styles of massage are: Swedish, Lymphatic, Rolphing (also goes by another name), Zone Therapy is a pressure point massage for the feet. It is amazing. Try it.

Meditation Therapy: There are so many types of meditation. But all of them encourage special music or no sound at all except for the sounds of the forest, the ocean, brook or whatever nature serves at the time of your meditation. If you are interested in music that will enhance your meditative state in a superb way, go to the web. www.centerpointe.com Empty your mind of all things. This used to be impossible for me. There were too many urgent duties to attend to. Keep at it. Allow thoughts to surface but do not dwell on any one thing for the moment. Relax and let the thoughts flow from one thought to another. When you are relaxed enough to feel that you are one with the ground, sand, bed, floor, couch, or chair, the thoughts are usually in a state of peaceful surrender. Now what you think of is usually what you need to act on in a confident way; in a committed way; in a safe way; in a loving way. Try reading books on meditation. You will gain such an insight.

Music Therapy: Some people who are disturbed or angry can not handle soothing angelic music. They thrive on music that fits the emotion they carry. This therapy should be done by a trained person. The individual receiving the therapy can choose certain songs that resonate. Let that person talk about the music: how it makes him/her feel, what it makes him/her feel like doing and what is he/she thinking etc. The therapist asks if he/she wants to feel that way. Play angelic music and watch the reactions. Turn it off if the recipient shows signs of stress or anger. Ask again how it makes

22

him/her feel, what it makes him/her feel like doing and what is he/she thinking etc. The therapist asks why he/she is feeling that way. Verbalizing and writing responses down are beneficial but it should depend on the recipient.

For someone who is not disturbed, you do not need a trained person. Lie back, empty your mind and let the music soak in. Visualize a retreat of your choice, sink into the moment and let your thoughts flow. You can write down afterwards what you thought and felt. Any song that will stir your soul will do. Some songs have sincere messages that duplicate your souls' desire. Heal the World, From a Distance, I Believe There are Angels Among Us, are songs for my soul.

Photo Therapy: There are a number of ways to do this therapy that are associated with photographs/pictures. Organize your photos to create a self history. Whether you have photos of yourself or not look through magazines. You can pick out photos of:
   a.   babies that may have looked like you
   b.   toddlers that may have looked like you
   c.   preteens that would have looked like you
   d.   things that you would have loved to do
   e.   things that you would have loved to have
Create a folder or pasteboard or even wall of pictures of who you would love to be. This is a form of age regression that is powerful.

You can use **Scrap Booking** or **Photo Max** to organize your pictures. I use Photo Max because it cost nothing to sign up and you can have all your pictures copied and saved on a secure website.

Another form of Photo/Picture Therapy is the same as the first except that you will be cutting out pictures of what you want now and who you want to be in the near future. The law of attraction as explained in the movie **"The Secret"** is very powerful. Watch the movie over and over. Each time you do, you will recognize how you have been using the principles and how much you can improve. This will encourage you to consistently improve.

Prayer Therapy: This is the one that is the most magical or better yet miraculous and yet so many people leave this one out. It is the most simple and yet is the one that is left until one is simply desperate. Desperate prayers do not work as fast as prayers that keep a continual line open to the higher source: Even God.

God is Love. God is also our creator. He not only IS love He loves. He loves enough to give us what we most desire even if going through extreme challenges gets us what we really want.

People abandon God but God will never abandon us.

Keep your communication open with Him and when you need something, He is faster to act.

Let's use the analogy of the computer. If you need to get online it takes a few minutes to get your computer up and running, and depending on what speed and equipment install you have, it takes you X number of minutes. If you are already online, it takes a fraction of the time. Stay online with God.

Rainbow Therapy: This can be done even if you do not experience any noticeable response. If you have little or no response and have a desire for immediate response, do your color therapy first. Get in a comfortable position and comfortable surrounding. Close your eyes. Picture a rainbow. The rainbow is a gift. This rainbow signifies love, acceptance, forgiveness, relationships and such. In your minds eye, picture you and the one you want to give this gift to, off in the distance. In your minds eye, toss the rainbow to the receiver. Notice if she/he catches the rainbow. If he/she does not catch it, there are walls or misgivings between you. Keep tossing the rainbow. Soon he/she will catch it. Sometimes giving a person a call will open the way for the recipient to receive it. The stronger your intention the sooner he/she will respond. Often it is caught the first time.

Rapid Eye Therapy: It is helpful to have other people assisting but not necessary. There are physical responses with this and many healing processes. Everybody is different. Possible responses are: crying, twisting, thrashing, yawning, coughing, laughing, and others

24

that appear to be wrenching out the traumas. Facilitator or assistant reminds recipient to blink and breathe, A pitcher of water is necessary for the recipient and the Facilitator. The breathing and blinking will release fears from the body and cells and the muscular response is an indication that it is happening. There are not always muscular responses such as crying, stretching, etc., but there should be a damp towel in case it is needed and a pillow for those who thrash.

There are 9 basic emotions that a person could have. They are:
1.   Rejection
2.   Control (loss of)
3.   Love (loss of)
4.   Not enough (money, time, friends etc)
5.   Health (lack of)
6.   Blame (loss of approval, decisions)
7.   Unfair
8.   Death
9.   Failure

The Facilitator repeats over and over while tapping on the temple negative statements which need to be squished out.

Normally I would never have a negative statement repeated over and over again. In this case we are taking the negative and eliminating it. Do not say these negatives. Let the Facilitator say it only while tapping so that you can squeeze it out involuntarily.

There are many stories about the benefits of RET (REM). This is one of the best forms of emotional release for many people. I have seen miracles.

Reiki Therapy: Reiki means universal energy or spiritual energy. The Reiki therapist is a conduit through which universal energy flows into the person who is being healed. Symbols are used and called symbols of light. To increase effectiveness, some therapists exhale a breathy sound as they give each symbol. Some people have a negative reaction to this. Some cultures call it "the Breath of Life." I say, "what ever works, works." It can be quite powerful. There are 12 levels. I have done all 12 levels which classifies me as a Reiki Master should I decide to practice again.

25

Script Therapy: There are a number of script therapies. I use the one created by Neil Voss. He let me name it "Release and Return." You basically acknowledge a weakness without putting blame or judgment on it and basically get rid of it. I was planning to share it with you in the book but realize that the first session needs to be done with a guide. I am a guide and have had much success with it. Everyone I have worked with has had results and some of them have been done over the phone. This approach covers your beliefs in all three areas: physical, mental, and feeling. 1. Say it very slowly. 2. Keep tapping your left palm on the lower right side with the 4 fingers of your right hand, 3. Read the script aloud for as many times as you need to, to feel the words flow through you. It usually takes from 3 to 20 times depending on how deep the issue is. Read slowly while tapping. Contact me if you would like to find out more.

Some feel this is more effective than Rapid Eye Therapy. I have used both methods. I value them both. You can do the script on your own when you are ready, after you have been instructed by a guide. The guide can do it over the phone. Both methods are life altering for the better.

Tap Therapy: The first time I became familiar with Tap Therapy was in or around 1990. I was traveling along interstate 80 at Donner Pass. The trip started out in Elk Grove, California at 4 or 5 in the morning. I was traveling by myself. My reasoning for starting at that time was because it would be late enough by the time I got to the Sierra Nevada Mountains after the ice had melted on the road. The journey was very pleasant and all the ice was melted until I rounded a bend at the peak of Donner Pass. There was a drop on the right side of thousands of feet and the left side was a mountain. When I hit the ice and started sliding I maneuvered toward the mountain. After I hit, I got out surveyed the damage. Luckily, I thought, I could make it to my destination being Provo, UT to pick up my son from College. My mental condition at the time, I didn't know. I was just obsessed with getting to my destination. When I arrived and packed my son's belongings, I couldn't get back in the truck. I was terrified. My cousin took me to a Chiropractor who practiced Tap Therapy. After the tapping session, the fear ceased and I was able to get back in my truck and head back to California.

26

Tapping is used for a number of other therapies as well: One being RET 'Rapid Eye Therapy'.

Writing Therapy: This can be done in a group with a guide or by simply going off by yourself and getting started. In a group the leader will ask a question. When that question is answered, the leader will ask another one. Quiet soothing music should be playing. The lights should be soft, dimmed a little as to ward off glare. If you are by yourself, get in a comfortable position and comfortable surroundings. Start writing. If your experiences, traumas and trials cause extreme emotion, stop writing until you have cried all your tears, or screamed all your screams or pounded until your strength gives out. Rest and resume when you have the strength. You may have to go through numerous episodes, so write and release as often as you need. The punch goes out of the experience. This is powerful.

Yoga Therapy and Table Yoga Therapy: If you have the strength for Yoga there are a few ways you can do it. Take a Yoga Class, go on a Yoga retreat or get a good Yoga book. Although Yoga doesn't look that difficult, it takes excellent balance and muscle strength to maintain those holds. Table Yoga is excellent for straightening out your back. With years of work requiring looking down a lot such as child care, cooking, lab assistance or technician, secretaries, teachers, lawyers, bookworms and others, gravity has a way of dragging you down. Use a massage table, firm bed or even a table that will hold your body, not your limbs. Others may like to go to the source: India

Yoga began in India with a few people who developed a way of handling the atrocities of their country. They never chose to be poor but because they were, it was important to find a way to deal with it. The people of India have made it a way of life without the name Yoga attached to it. They do the deep breathing concentration and meditation in their homes while the westerners and a few easterners make it a big to-do. Easterners gear Yoga to their own individual needs. They may get a teacher for a few months to learn and practice what they need individually and then when learned, continue to do it on their own. For many, Yoga is always very much part of the family fitness routine.

A western movement came alive in the 60's. Westerners sought the eastern way of music and Yoga and brought it to the west. At first, easterners who had an aversion to the hippie and cult thing looked at westerners and thought they were nuts. Now it is the people with the money who are seeking this unique experience.

Yoga began to flourish in the west because of the interest of the west in the ways of the east; however, the depth and the knowledge is believed to be best experienced in the east; India.

It was the western influence that caused a sweep of interest in Yoga.

If you wish to do Table Yoga at home, use a table or firm bed and lie on your stomach with your head and arms hanging over the side. Let your body stretch then twist with gravity, Keep stretching and twisting at every angle you can think of and then turn on you back and do the same thing. As each muscle pulls and pulls and pulls, it will release stress and you will be able to stretch that much more and limber up your body. It is fun and so relaxing. You can fall asleep afterwards for more healing or you might feel so rejuvenated that you may want to get up and get that project done, be it work or play.

There are ways in which you can check with your inner knowing to learn what will work best for you and who you can work well with. One is by muscle testing and another one is by using a pendulum. This needs to be taken seriously if you want the best results. If you ask questions that are none of your business, don't expect to get accurate answers. I did not use these methods as a "sealed in stone" answer. It was more of a support.   I asked God the question and sometimes checked with a pendulum.   This proved to be more accurate for me than the muscle testing. Muscle testing just does not work if you are dehydrated or not electrical. The index finger is the yes finger, the middle finger is the no finger and the thumb is the uncertain finger. Hold the pendulum over the yes finger and say "Yes." See which way the pendulum swings. Hold the pendulum over the no finger and say "No." See which way the pendulum swings. Over the thumb, say "not discernable", This will happen if you have a two part question or if the question doesn't make sense or you do not need to know. When you become more decisive and your natural knowing, intuition or inspiration is strong, you will have no need for this. You will just know. I no longer need this.

28

SECTION ONE
CHAPTER THREE
HEALING ACTIVITIES

There are a number of indications that a therapy is working for you. Most of them have a squeezing or repelling action as to expel all the old air from the system such as coughing, laughing, yawning, crying, stretching and thrashing, among others. After you squish the issues from within you, you will probably feel very tired. Lie down and sleep. That is when your body heals faster. Drink a glass of pure water before you sleep. Your body spends a lot of energy digesting food and cuts down the healing process. For best results, do not eat before you sleep and Do Drink Water.

Some people who have worked through their issues may not react in these ways but still get great benefits

If you are working with someone to assist in doing emotional release ask if they want the light dimmed. Sometimes a person can not release if they feel uncomfortable with someone looking at them. Make sure they are in a comfortable position and comfortable temperature.

Affirmations: Affirmations assist in reprogramming your subconscious belief system, and eventually your conscious. If you find yourself arguing with a positive affirmation, try asking the question. Example: I am happy. (Bologna), that's a big lie etc, etc, etc.) Try saying each of these sentences a number of times until you don't feel like arguing. First, "Am I happy?" "Maybe I'm happy." "I'm going to be happy." "I think I am happy." Then try "I Am Happy!"

If you listen to subliminal messages in the background of music over and over while you are awake or while you sleep, you cannot argue with the messages and they will be faster and easier to accept. You can create your own affirmations or use existing ones. I have created 3 sets of affirmations for the following subjects: Learning/Testing, Health & Fitness, Prosperity and Abundance. Subliminal messages are statements which you don't consciously perceive with your senses but are received by your subconscious mind. Hundreds of research studies prove that the subconscious mind absorbs stimulus that is missed by the conscious mind. During your life, you have absorbed many, if not myriads of negative statements. Positive affirmations are a most powerful tool in changing subconscious thought into positive thoughts and actions and even a state of being. The subconscious mind is very powerful. It affects the very things we do without thinking. In a sense it affects the very essence of who we are. Within this music there are hundreds of positive affirmations that reach the subconscious mind, and have a strong influence on your conscious actions, thoughts, habits, and behaviors that make up who you are and how you experience life. These help negate the negative. Many of the affirmations are repeated within each CD to reinforce the positive.

If you decide to create your own affirmations make sure you use "I am" often, as it is powerful in and of itself.

Brain integration: It is important to have the left brain and right brain integrated. There are a number of ways to achieve this: Any activity that physically crosses over the center of your body. This is good for mental stress and can be done before studying, homework or tests. Each exercise should be about 30 seconds.

1. Place your pointer finger and middle finger together in the center of the forehead, press firmly and rub your fingers back and forth briskly with your eyes closed.
2. Hold your hands together, hold them up above head (not over head) and simply put 'do a figure 8'. Clap your hands in any sound pattern and alternate with each side of the body" Left right left right and so on.
3. Beat on your chest with your knuckles or fingers of both hands. Left hand on left side and Right hand on right side. Alternate left and right. Imitate a gorilla.
4. Run or walk with each leg crossing over the other leg as you go.

There are many other activities you can do that will work if the activity crosses your left arm or leg to the right side and cross your right arm or leg to the left side. I used brain integration on students with dyslexia and they had increased performance in their homework, testing, and ultimately their grades went up.

The music from Centerpointe Technologies Institute is excellent for brain integration as well as meditation. You can get it on their web site at **www.centerpoint.com**

Cleansing: We covered one type of cleansing in the hydro-therapy information. That is Colon Therapy. Having a clean colon makes it very improbable for one to get the diseases connected to the colon. There are a number of other cleanses: liver cleanse, gall bladder cleanse, detoxification cleanse and bacteria cleansing, to name a few.

I did a gall bladder cleanse. The gall stones turned into rubber-like balls and passed painlessly. I fasted for a few days and did an enema to eliminate everything I could before the cleanse. Since I was pretty much empty, the gall stones were visible as they passed with the enema water.

Some people shy away from enemas and high colonics. I'm just the opposite. I'll do just about anything to get rid of the toxins (poisons) and putrefied fecal matter. The benefits are so astounding that people look forward to the process in anticipation of feeling better and sometimes actually feeling good. A popular use for the enema is to bring down a fever really fast.

Some people are turning to raw food. This is a good way to cleanse the colon, but it is still a good idea to get a colonic irrigation now and then. It assists in making it so your intestines are clean and functioning correctly.

Coloring: This is covered in section one. It is very relaxing so just have fun and do it.

Detoxifying: Soak in water/bleach or water/vinegar in the bathtub. Fill the bath tub just high enough to cover you. Only 2 or 3 capfuls of bleach or vinegar is enough. Soak for approximately 20 to 40 minutes. Bring a good book with you or put on some relaxing music. Close your eyes and take deep breaths and blow it out all the way.

Exercising: This is covered in Section one. It is very rejuvenating so just have fun and do it.

Fasting: Fasting gives your system a rest. It needs a rest at least once a month for 24 hours. Any amount will help. Drink 4 ounces of water every time you think of it. Water should be pure. If you drink distilled water as some suggest, it is imperative that you add mineral water to it. Otherwise drink purified. Depletion of minerals can be dangerous.

Fasting eliminates toxins from the system. Do not fast for long periods of time if you are extremely toxic. Drink water continually. Add cleansing herbs for long fasts. The second night is when you start dropping larger amounts of toxins and it is extremely hard on the heart to have toxins rushing through it without water and cleansing herbs to help carry out the toxins.

Feng-shui: This trigram has been westernized to fit into the western lifestyle. This BA-Gua Map is to be used over a floor plan.

BA-GUA MAP

Abundance Energy (Wealth) Purple (secondary Red & Blue) Late Spring Air, Wind, Wood, Water	External Recognition (Fame) Red Summer Fire	Intimacy (commitment) Silver, Pink Late Summer Fall Earth
Ancestors/protectors (Origin of) Green Spring Wood	Health Yin and Yang Heaven & Earth Yellow, Brown Never ending cycle of life Earth	Creativity (Children, Ideas) White, Rainbow Autumn Metal
Self-knowledge (Wisdom) Blue, Brown Early Spring Big Earth (Mountain)	Journey (Career) Black/Dark Blue Winter Water	Helpful people Mentors (Travel, Spirit, Community) Grey/Silver Late Fall Heaven/Metal

Each square box above will be referred to as a center after this. Decide what you would want in your centers. Here are some suggestions.

As you walk through the door, look to your far left. That is the Wealth Center. The color is purple, red and blue. The element is air, wind, wood and water. In the wealth Center you could have an aquarium, water fall or anything that has the colors and elements.

Straight ahead to the furthest wall is the Fame Center. This is a good place for a fire place or red candles or even a picture with the color, element and rising shape-like triangle, such as a sale boat.

To your far right is the Commitment Center. Doubles should go there. Pictures of couples: wedding, parents, two trees, two cows, etc., a shelf with two teddy bears, two dolls, two vases, two statues or whatever.

To the left midway is the Ancestors Center and there can be pictures of your ancestors, pictures of the country where your ancestor originated and use the colors and elements. Wood frames with green matt board, decorated piece with drift wood and green plant life. There are other things you can have in this center that symbolizes protectors. Different people have different symbols for protection. Dragons are for China and US. The Inca has three: Bird, snake and cat.

In the center of the room is the Health Center. Earth is brown; Wood is brown; brown floors, brown coffee table, brown bed, brown table. A young boy was always sick. The mother decided to try yellow on the boys' bed. In a matter of a few days the boys' health increased.

To the right, midway is the Creativity/Children's Center: Use the colors white and rainbow and the element is metal. Have your creative ideas there along with children and family.

If your door enters the room on the left side, you are entering at the Wisdom Center. If you enter the room in the center, you are entering the career center. If you are entering the room on the right side, you are entering in the Mentor Center.

If a window or door is in one of your centers, hang something from the ceiling or place a rug on the floor at the door.

The Wisdom Center is on the left as you enter the door. Use the colors blue, brown and the earth/mountain is element of this center. Books of wisdom can go here.

The Career Center is in the center as you enter the door. It should have something that pertains to your career and, of course, use the color black and/or dark blue. The water element is with this center.

The Mentor/Helpful people Center is on the right as you enter the door. It is also known as the Travel/Fun Center. You can have anyone you admire including God, Jesus Christ, Buddha, Mohamad, Angels, spiritual activities, prayer poems and pictures, and travel plans.

If you have a talent or career that you would like to receive wealth, fame or success in, put it in that center. If it is your career, put it in as many centers as you wish. If you want wealth, fame and success in your career, put it in all three centers. A photographer would put it in the Wealth Center, Fame Center and Career Center. Even the Creative Center would work.

There is so much more information about Feng-shui, but the last one I wish to mention is the flow of energy. If your front door and back door are in direct alignment, and both doors are open and the air rushes in and rushes out, this is not good Feng-shui. Put a hanging plant or floor plant to block the sudden breeze that comes through. Hang a crystal from the ceiling to block the sudden flow. Good energy is vital

If you have clutter in your home, it blocks good Feng-shui. There is so much and it is almost impossible to do it all so do what you think, and feel is fun: something that uplifts the soul.

If the home is not square certain energies of the home are not present. There is a way around that. You can use the whole building plan and/or each room. I have focused on rooms. You can do the same for your house. It takes a little more doing if your house is not square but it can be done with tricks. If you want more detail, there are plenty of books on Feng-shui. This is just to familiarize you with it so you can decide if you want to go deeper.

Silent Witness: Wayne Dyer calls it Silent Witness. It is almost like stepping out of the scene and watching what is happening to you from the audience or from a distance. The first time I experienced this, it was amazing. I was being yelled at, degraded and accused. I watched the man's mouth open and close and heard a pattern of sounds and didn't even feel any emotion. The man wore down and I got up and walked away.

In the Juvenile Service System, we had training on how to de-escalate an irate youth or parent. I was in the position twice to de-escalate but I was doing it without noticing. I truly cared about the parent in each case and listened (silent witness type) with no emotion of my own, just understanding the emotions of the parent. After they were listened to I gave feedback. "I can assure you that these counselors love your son." I said it with commitment and with the power of intention. In both cases, the parent became grateful for the positive and was able to better handle the negative.

Touch for health: This is a system that is not called "therapy" but truly is a Therapy: Your body is a magnet of sorts. North and south magnetism emit from alternate fingers and the palms of the hands and feet emit powerful energy enough to create a proper balance.

In China, a doctor is paid for keeping a person healthy. Here in the U.S. a doctor gets paid when a patient is sick.

In China, there is a way to know if a person will get sick within a 6 month period. There are 12 meridians in your body, not too much unlike electricity. If there is a short or break in your electric current the appliance malfunctions. The same is true of the meridians of your body. It is fairly simple to balance out the meridians. The magnetism in your hands, when run across the body in the correct pattern for each meridian will balance it. Major stress can bump it out of balanced alignment. People who have "Healing Hands" either know what they are doing or they are simply "inspired." I will cover stress in another portion of my book.

The power of intention: Wayne Dyer has a book with this title. Good book. Good reading for anyone, and anyone can accomplish their goals by putting it to use. If your intention is clear, that "you will be well", you will find the therapies and procedures that are best for you, and you will be well. The scriptures call it faith. If you fully intend for it to happen, you will have the faith and it will happen.

The Native American Way: Most ethnic groups have a way of healing and receiving guidance from the world around them.

First the healing way: A group of about 40 or 50 of us met in the Utah wilderness to experience survival techniques from a Native American leader. We learned how to get water out of the ground, how to make various types of tents from trees and brush. We learned which trees and bark were used to make them well and make them sick. My purpose is to let you know that things out there exist and it is wonderful to experience the different ways of different people

The book "Medicine Cards" by Jaimie Sams & David Carson makes it easy to understand how the Native Americans learned from their animal guides. The book describes what each animal represents. It is very interesting and fun. My animal guides were picked. I noticed how they really did represent my talents, goals and desires. The knowing and feeling was like, "of course, I knew that." It was like an eye opener. Good fun stuff.

SECTION ONE
CHAPTER FOUR
DEVICES OF WELL BEING

The government has a tight reign on devices and products that claim to heal. The law was created because merchants many years ago would do a fast emotional sell and skip town before people realized they had been taken. The emotional state of people in dire need for health is weakened by desperation and they may try anything to get relief. Some of this is basic information that you already know. The following are devices and products, people feel made a difference in their lives as far as health is concerned. The truth is that nothing really heals the body except the body and the mind. Other things only assist the body in healing.

What you already know is that we all need oxygen via the air we breathe, oxygenated and nutrient blood in our veins, and nutrition and oxygen in our cells. Most of us do not know the exact balance of which nutrients.

The way most of us find out what is good for us is by trial and error. Even the doctors say "Let's try this medication. If this doesn't work we'll try something else." They can pretty well guess because of the studies and education they have been through. But it is not without failures. If you purchase a medication, you do not get your money back. You do not get your money back when you see a doctor. On the other hand you do have 72 hours to change your mind in case of a high pressured sales person when you purchase a wellness product or device or the 15-30 day trials offered by some companies.

If there was a product that would assist in oxygenation or blood circulation throughout your body or assist in eliminating poisonous garbage that might attack your body in different ways, would you be interested? Many people experience relief from many forms of maladies after using devices and products that are not offered by doctors. The AMA and FDA have tight control over doctors and what they can do. I know doctors who have lost their license because they were providing for their patients products that were out of the realm of prescribed medicine even though their patients were overcoming dis-ease. I go to a doctor when they can assist me in their area of expertise never expecting them to cross over to an alternative route. I wouldn't put them through that disharmony.

Doctors in other countries are the exception. In China a doctor doesn't get paid unless his patient is healthy. In Japan doctors have the freedom to use what makes a person well. In the U.S., doctors are paid when a patient is sick, then they give medicine which covers up the symptoms and produces other side effects or symptoms.

Assists in Healing
Crystals: Crystals are an excellent way to hold a positive energy. Whether you have your crystals programmed or not, they are a great benefit. When you acquire a crystal, you may want to clear the energy of the crystal by soaking in salt water for 24 hours and then rinsing it with cold water. If you do not program the crystal, it will magnify the energy of its surroundings. If there is peace and harmony in your home, it will multiply that peace and harmony. If there is contention, it will magnify that. We have never programmed our crystals; however, we have felt certain vibrations from them and accepted them. One is my healing crystal. I put it on my chest when I have a cold and the cold is gone in the morning. One, gives off the feeling of confidence and strength or power. To program a crystal, cleanse and rinse it first and then clear any negative feelings and hold the crystal and focus whatever energy you want into the crystal such as: Love, power, peace, harmony, success or strength. You can mix two energies if they go together like peace and harmony, freedom and joy, love and laughter.

Rough, uncut stones often posses a far greater energy than those that have been cut and polished.

Chi Machine
The # 1 healing system in Japan is The Chi machine and Hot House. The Chi Machine oxygenates the body.
The spinal influence on health: Within the brain and extending through the core of the spinal column is the central nervous system

and branching out from it is the nerve network that reaches every part of the body and provides all body functioning not under conscious control such as breathing, digestion, heart rate etc. This extended nerve network is termed the Autonomic Nervous System and it further divides into the Sympathetic and Parasympathetic Nervous Systems which provide vital balance to the body's nerve functioning. Any impairment to the spinal alignment or abnormal spinal pressure on vertebrae joints can impair the autonomic nervous system resulting in minor and major body dysfunction, disorder and disease. The spinal column bone marrow is also a source of blood production and immune system globulin upon which middle aged adults are more dependent, following depletion of globulin production from the commonly aged and shrinking thymus gland.

Utilization of full spinal movement: The spine's design permits sideways snake-like movement that serves to relieve vertebrae joint pressure and thereby promote greater well being. The Chi Machine delivers the best possible lateral snake-like movement to the spine with the body in the ideal therapeutic position. When the massage concludes you may experience the therapeutic benefit of a sensation similar to that of yawning and stretching.

Four main features of the Chi Machine are:
1. Full body exercise with no side effect
2. Just lie down to use it, there is no effort or stress involved
3. No injury
4. Simple, comfortable and easy to develop a regular exercise habit

Six major benefits derived for using the Chi Machine:
1. Cellular Activation
2. Spinal Balancing
3. Improving the Immune System
4. Blood Production
5. Restoration of Balance to the Autonomic Nervous System
6. Exercising Internal Organs

HOT HOUSE: Far Infrared Rays (FIR) are emitted from the hot house. Within the magnetic spectrum, some rays, such as light, can be seen by the unaided human eye. Most, however, are totally invisible to us. FIR are well beyond the ability of the naked eye to see. FIR is capable of penetrating deep into the human body. It can gently and delightfully elevate the body's temperature to 99f. When it does so, it helps to expand capillaries which stimulate blood circulation. This increases the body's energy reserve and accelerates the metabolic exchange between blood and body tissue. FIR can actually increase the body tissue's regenerative ability and gives the body a feeling of well being, Blood circulation increases, metabolism is improved and internal organs are stimulated.

MAGNETIC THERAPY DEVICES: Devices that are effortless are my favorite. I am not sure who the others are but Nikken is a company that I know of that offers magnetic devices and they have good products. They carry both magnetic and far infrared ray products. Magnetic Therapy is believed to be a temporary one because the magnetic energy that heals is guided to a particular part of the body which can weaken another part or parts of the body. Therefore, use the magnets in a place of pain or injury and remove the magnets until the next injury. The first product they came out with 30 years ago was a magnetic bed pad. This sleeping system gives most people the energy for tomorrow while you sleep tonight. Sounder sleep and the ability to recuperate from fatigue more rapidly are the results of this unique sleep system. They have added a comforter with FIR included. A magnetic seat pad is for those who sit for long periods of time and need to feel more rested as they work or drive. Mag steps were also offered 30 years ago and since then Nikken has added numerous other products that can increase wellness. I got mine when they first came out and discovered that I got up in the morning feeling rested and invigorated with a calm stomach. There is one thing that is important to know. Not everyone is a candidate for this sleep system. If you sleep with a partner it is possible that one or the other of you will not have the same response. We discovered that was the case with my husband and me, so I just use it for napping periodically if I feel under the weather. I find, I no longer need it.

Theoretically, if disease can not live in an oxygenated system, it stands to reason that getting oxygen to all parts of the body is essential. The faster, further and the more rocks the water hits in a brook, the purer the water. Likewise, when the blood rushes through the body with the aid of magnetization, there is great benefit.

I like products that I do not have to think about. With a good sleep system, a good air filter and a good water system I have 3 things I do not have to think about. It is necessary that I go to sleep every night on a bed. The investment is crucial if rest is crucial. I know what it is like to be a semi-invalid. Sleeping on a magnetic bed took me to a new level of health. I have since made other discoveries such as **Layers of Light** that will be covered later.

One word of caution on Magnets: Do not try to concoct your own magnetic devices. Magnets can be harmful if the wrong gauss is used. If the magnetic field of the earth is duplicated it should be just fine. If the magnetic device is a little stronger than the Magnetic Field of the earth, which should also be fine considering the magnetic field of the earth is less than it was when people lived nearly a thousand years. Since Magnetic energy has a positive and a negative, if your home is like the majority of homes that have more positive energy because of all the electrical currents, you need to balance with a negative magnetic field which is usually more beneficial. **Layers of Light** has a system whereby we can be protected from the Electro Magnetic Field and much more.

For health's sake, if you can sleep comfortably out doors, that is generally magnetically balanced and oxygen rich and the best way to sleep.

If that is not possible, what really matters is that you get a good night's sleep, but a good night sleep is not all you need. The type of persons I have noticed who do not particularly benefit from the magnetic devices are people who are already high energy people. But if you can trust Nikken's scientific approach to magnetic healing take a serious look at it.

42

Environment: Nikken Air Wellness™ Power5™:Daily exposure to indoor air pollution can be as much as 100 times higher than to polluted air outside. The Nikken Power5 can make breathing indoors more enjoyable because it combines advanced air filtration with negative-ion generation and aromatherapy technology. Its HEPA filter meets the standard used in laboratories and hospital operating rooms. Five separate stages of filtration reduce a wide range of air contaminants. Only the Nikken Power5 uses all major filtration methods to create clean air without creating emission byproducts. An exclusive Nikken technology, clean ion generation, produces negative ions without creating ozone. And only the Power5 adds a selectable aromatherapy system — a natural, effortless, non-invasive means of promoting wellness through relaxation and stress reduction. The Air Wellness Power5 is designed for fully automated operation, with sensors that activate it when changes in air quality are detected. It is also supplied with a convenient remote control, and includes energy-saving features. With the Power5, you can experience the air you were meant to breathe, every day.

Nikken PiMag™ Water System: Discovered near a small town in Japan more than 30 years ago, pi water is called "the water of life" by scientists. Created by natural mineral deposits and negative ions, pi water has been duplicated in the laboratory — and the result is the Nikken PiMag Water System. This system has highly sophisticated filtration technology. But it is more than a filter. Special pi ceramics from deep-sea coral reflect far-infrared energy — sometimes called the "wavelength of life." The water flows through a magnetic field to complete the process. With the PiMag Water System, delicious water is available instantly, whenever you turn the tap. And because it is right from your faucet, it's more convenient and less expensive than bottled water. Best of all, it's PiMag water - the water of life.

The Nikken PiMag Optimizer II is specifically designed to produce water your body needs. The Optimizer features a pi ring of special coral that comes from the deep ocean. This ring contains calcium carbonate, a mineral used in Japan as a natural way to modify water's acid/alkaline balance. Powerful rotating magnets produce a complex magnetic field, and the vortex action adds oxygen. In minutes, you have optimized water for drinking, cooking, any use.

Those who try it report that it tastes "lighter" and more refreshing than ordinary water. Find out how good your drinking water can be!

Nikken PiMag™ Aqua Pour: Using an ingenious gravity flow system, the PiMag Aqua Pour can provide you with Nikken PiMag water no matter where you are. It's a portable waterworks — producing PiMag water without electricity or plumbing. The Aqua Pour features several stages of filtration, including carbon, ion exchange resin and zeolite. Pi ceramics are in the filter, to impart "the water of life." Final stage filtration consists of mineral stones, and Nikken Magnetic Technology completes the process. It's the most convenient way to have a supply of PiMag water at home, in the office, while traveling - practically anywhere.

Although there are great water systems that make a big difference in our quality of water, it is necessary to purchase filters periodically and you need units for a number of different areas such as the sink, the shower and wherever you want good water.

I was introduced to The Bon Aqua System which is a whole house and yard system that I researched and found to be a remarkable system. The Bon Aqua Water System cleans and purifies the complete water system in your home and yard without harmful chemicals and without maintenance and filters to purchase. It saves a lot of work, space, money and health. I prefer the system for the whole house and yard so that my garden can grow better, eliminate stains in my bathroom and kitchen and have all the pipes in my house clean and void of disease causing toxins; This unit cleans pipes with no harmful chemicals and no filters to buy and no upkeep. There is actual proof this System works. See back of book for e-mail address and more information.

I lost contact with my connection. If you hear of it elsewhere I highly recommend it for those who want really clean germ free pipes.

Since there is new technology being discovered almost daily, it is good to stay informed.

SECTION ONE
CHAPTER FIVE
PRODUCTS OF WELL BEING

Essential Oils: The following is some research I have found on essential oils: Essential Oils are believed to be man's first medicine. The use of oils are documented in hieroglyphics. There are 188 references to oils in the Bible. An archeological expedition discovered and oil distillery in a monastery in Egypt. When digging, a wall collapsed. Five alabaster jars with essential oils were found. They still have full frequency. A vase was also found that contained tree scrolls, one's author is believed to be Jesus and one is believed to be Mary Magdalene. In the two years they have been examined by the British Museum, all Tests are confirming their validity. They describe the use of essential oils in healing.

Whether this is true or not, essential oils are said to have measurements in kilohertz (electrical) energy and vibration rates that boost the health and well being of we humans. I understand John Hopkins has a study on this subject. What we do know is that the higher the frequency, energy, and vibratory rate, the healthier we are mentally and physically.

Essential oils can help us raise our frequency.

Disease cannot exist in an oxygen rich environment. Oxygen delivers nutrients to the blood. You must get nutrients into the cell. Cells mutate with as little as a 1% drop in oxygen in the serum around the cell. There are 5 stages of mutation, the fifth being cancer.

Essential oils are catalysts. They are lipid soluble and can immediately penetrate the cell wall to bring oxygen and nutrients into the cell.

For a list of essential oils and what they are historically used for, see Aroma Therapy on page 7.

FOOD STATE
Health Discoveries by R. Neil Voss
This research backs up Food State's usage of Vitamins

Sherlock Holmes said "when you have examined all the logical possibilities and have not found the answer, you should look for the most unobvious solution, regardless of how illogical it may be." Look for an unobvious solution, regardless of how unorthodox it may be.

The Health and Nutrition Examination Survey found:
1. 45 % of the population ate no fruits, vegetables, and drank no juice.
2. 27% had no fruit
3. 22% had no vegetables
4. 29% had 2 servings of fruit
5. 27% had 2 servings of fruits and vegetables

It is recommended that we get 5-9 fruits and vegetable in our diet. What did you have today?

"Biochemist Harold N. Simpson states, *"There is starvation in America. This type of starvation is not due to insufficient food but deficiency of needed food elements in food. Nutritive shortages such as vitamin and mineral deficits cannot be fixed by a vitamin pill consisting of chemical-isolated vitamins. Whole foods contain all related nutrients; vitamins, minerals, trace minerals enzymes, co-enzymes, amino acids, fatty acids, and factors that function together for the biochemical equilibrium of the human body."*

For example, HGH starts to decline at about age 25 or earlier if you have a poor diet. By age 60 the average person only has 25%- 40% of normal. It takes 191 combinations of amino acids and lots of combinations of polysaccharides for your body to create HGH. HGH increases the speed of healing and repair and the rehabilitation of any damage.

"Clinical Studies on natural HGH show improved bone mineralization, reduced osteoporosis, increased heart and kidney function, good HDL, improved metabolic function, reduced triglycerides, improved immune function. HGH rebuilds all the organs, such as the bowel lining, skin, kidneys, eyes, and heart. It even repairs the damaged myelin found in neurodegenerative

46

diseases such as Alzheimer's, ALS, MS, fibromyalgia, diabetes, and others. There are 83 known human growth hormones. They tell the cells to accept nutrients, they help you lose fat and wrinkles, repair damage of age-related degeneration and even create new internal organs."

"Cellular function relies on correctly formed cell receptors. Eighty-six diseases have been linked to malformed receptors. Growth hormone must have intact receptors to attach to on cells in order for the cells to accept nutrients and repair or grow, or healing and growth is not going to happen.

Infections use receptor sites to attach to your cells; white blood cells (immune system) use receptor sites to identify and attack the infections."

"HGH must have intact receptors to attach to on cells in order for the cells to accept nutrients and repair or grow, or healing and growth is not going to happen, even in the presence of the correct nutrients. Through oral supplementation there are indications that deficiencies can be corrected and health built up until the body begins again to make correctly formed receptors from glycoproteins. [Glycoproteins are proteins combined with polysaccharides, or long-chained sugars]."

Our goal is to enable you to **compensate for toxic substances in your life, both physical and mental,** and to enable you to **enhance your physical, mental, and psychological performance** with these technological products and protocols.

These bioavailable products increase absorption resulting in *absoring 5 times more nutrients* in the blood and liver, *utilizing 16 times more nutrients*, enabling the cells to *retain nutrients 16 times longer.* On examination, these products **show a significantly *higher biological activity*, *requiring fewer products*, and having *greater results*.**

The carrier Protein has nutrients in addition to the vitamins and minerals not found in regular vitamins and minerals. They are loaded with amino acids, about 40% protein, full of polysaccharides (beta-glucans 1,3/1,6, & mannons), SOD, glutathione precursors, trace minerals, lipoic acid, B complex vitamins including B6, B12, GABA, more than 40 proteolytic enzymes, B 1 necessary for normal metabolism of carbohydrates and fats, biotin, nicotinic acid, pantothenate, folic acid, B6, Vitamin K, Zinc, Chromium, riboflavin", and much more according to Clinical Research. " Food State nutrients have a profound effect on E. Coli, salmonella, staphylococcus, and candida albicans, helping to eradicate them from the intestinal system." **How can we not include all these nutrients?**

"Vitamins only work with Coenzymes. Vitamins do not work unless they are complex to protein chaperone components. They are further enhanced when synergistically combined with enzymes, coenzymes, phyto-nutrients and trace element activators in a proper organic state."

COMPARISON of NUTRIENTS (per gram)

Vitamin/Minerals:	A	B1	B12	C	Zinc	Manganese	Chromium
Unit of Measure	IU	mcg	mcg	mg	mg	mg	mcg
Spirulina	2,300	31	3	0.05	0.03	0.05	2.8
Chlorella	555	17	1.3	0.1	0.70		
Wheat Grass	500	3	0.3	3.1	0.05	0.10	
Food State	250,000	250,000	5,000	250	50	50	2,000

* Research resulting from Clinical Studies

How can you compensate for the harmful effects of a poor lifestyle diet & diabetes?

"The reaction of glucose and other reducing sugars (short chain sugars) with protein is called "glycation." Glycation produces products which can easily break down to the starting materials, namely sugars and proteins. However, over a long period of time and due to the glycation products become irreversible, meaning that they no longer break down into protein and sugar. This irreversible reaction eventually damages the tissues and deactivates enzymes like SOC (Super Oxide Dismutase)."

"In two Clinical double blind, placebo studies with Food State Vitamin C and Food State Selenium were individually evaluated for their effect on glycation. Food State Vitamin C had decreased the amount of "glycation end products" by 46.8%. Food State Vitamin C was 68% more absorbed at 4 hours after ingestion and was more gradually absorbed than ascorbic acid alone. The majority of the subjects excreted less (120) Food State Vitamin C, whereas the ones who consumed ascorbic acid alone excreted more ascorbic acid (180), indicating that more was utilized by the Food State subjects. The author concludes that bioflavonoids, enzymes, and other co-factors in Food State Vitamin C are responsible for increased utilization." (Vinson, J.A., Bose, P., American Journal of. Clinical. Nutrition 48:601-604

"Food State Selenium decreased the amount of "glycation end products" by 75%. Food State Selenium is 123 times more effective in preventing non-enzymatic glycation than regular Selenium. Food State C is 35.3 times more effective than Vitamin B, and 16.5 times more effective than regular vitamin E." (Vinson, J.A., Howard, T. B., peer reviewed journal: Nutritional Biochemistry 7:659-663.)

Regular Isolate vitamins, minerals, and nutrients are toxic. These Food State nutrients are significantly lower toxicity than other nutritional products by Clinical Studies. For example, Food State Selenium is 300% less toxic than regular Selenium. (See Law Suit by Other Vitamin and Mineral Supplement Companies.)

Notice: This information is not intended to replace an order of a relationship with a qualified health care professional and is not intended as medical advice. This is intended as shared knowledge and information from research as stated above. The researcher encourages you to make your own health care decisions based upon your research and in partnership with a qualified health care professional.

We have a questionnaire available upon request in which the results will reveal to you an awareness of issues related to your quest for health.

The most productive, effective, and bio-available whole food products relating to these areas are available to you at your request. There is more information in the following pages on minerals.

Goji
This is the research R. Neil Voss learned from Goji

If you could take a drink a day, that makes you feel good, look good, lose weight, increases your energy, gets rid of all your stress and anxiety, and puts a silly grin on your face all day long, would you drink it?... I think the answer is yes!!! Everybody wants to experience these benefits! Free Life is a company that offers Goji drink that phenomenal and delicious. This is my favorite drink and it does just that for many people, me included. It is desired by so many people because of the taste and it probably is the most nutrient dense natural nutrition product ever discovered. The Himalayan Goji juice distributed by Free Life is a high frequency natural berry juice that out performs all else. It is jam packed with antioxidants, amino acids, polysaccharides, and many other nutrients which have been shown to promote many health benefits, vitality, energy, endurance, longevity, restful sleep, and a general sense of calm and well being.

Himalayan Goji Berry Juice: "The Most Nutrient Dense Nutrition Product I have seen in 40 years." – Dr Earl Mindell. The BEST that Nature has to Offer! It has a 3,000-year history in China and the East. This revered Berry has an annual two-week festival in its honor! The Chinese have been growing this alkaline fruit for thousands of years!

The Chinese hold a strong belief that this fruit can significantly extend life. The people of Ningxia Province in China, where these berries grow, are rumored to live up to 120 or even 150 years. The most well documented case of extreme longevity is the life of Li Qing Yuen who lived to the age of 252. He was born in the year 1678 and died in 1930. Li Qing Yuen gave a lecture at the University of Beijing at the age of 200. He consumed Goji daily as his primary food and was married 14 times and had 11 generations of posterity when he died in 1930. The life of Li Qing Yuen is the most well documented case of extreme longevity known.

- Goji berries contain up to 21 trace minerals (The main ones being zinc, iron, copper, calcium, germanium, selenium, and phosphorus).
- Goji berries are the richest source of carotenoids, including beta-carotene (more beta carotene than carrots), of all known foods or plants on earth!
- They contain 500 times the amount of vitamin C, by weight, than oranges making them second only to camu camu berries as the richest vitamin C source on earth.
- Goji berries also contain vitamins B1, B2, B6, and vitamin E.
- Mature fruits contain about 11 mg of iron per 100 grams, beta-sisterol (an anti-inflammatory agent), linoleic acid (a fatty acid), sesquiterpenoids (cyperone, solavetivone), tetraterpenoids (zeaxanthin, physalin), and betaine (0.1%).
- Goji berries contain 22 types of polysaccharides of which 4 are unique to the Goji berry. Polysaccharides have been found to fortify the immune system. One polysaccharide found in this fruit has been found to be a powerful secretagogue (a substance that stimulates the secretion of rejuvenative human growth hormone by the pituitary gland).
- Goji berries have been traditionally regarded as a longevity, strength building, and sexual potency food of the highest order. In several study groups with elderly people the berry was given once a day for 3 weeks, many beneficial results were experienced and 67% of the patients T cell transformation functions tripled and the activity of the patient's white cell interleukin-2 doubled. In addition, the results showed that all the patients spirit and optimism increased significantly, appetite improved in 95% of the patients, 95% of the patients slept better, and 35% of the patients partially recovered their sexual function.
- There are many other nutrients too numerous to mention!

Here are 34 reasons Goji Juice is supreme according to Freelife

1. Extends life, protecting the body from premature aging through its powerful antioxidant action
2. Increases energy and strength, especially when fighting disease
3. Makes people feel and look younger. **Goji** stimulates the secretion of **HGH** (human growth hormone) the "youth hormone."
4. Maintains healthy blood pressure
5. Reduces the risk of cancer
6. Reduces cholesterol
7. Promotes normal blood sugar in early adult-onset diabetes
8. Enhances sexual function and treats sexual dysfunction
9. Helps weight reduction
10. Relieves headaches and dizziness
11. Relieves insomnia and improves the quality of sleep
12. Supports eye health and improves your vision
13. Strengthens the heart
14. Inhibits lipid **peroxidation** (a cause of heart disease)
15. Improves disease resistance
16. Improves immune response (T-cell, IL-2, **IgA, IgG**)
17. Cancer treatment
18. Restores and repairs DNA (preventing mutations that can cause cancer)
19. Inhibits tumor growth
20. Reduces the toxic effects of chemotherapy and radiation
21. Builds strong blood, enhancing production of red blood cells, white blood cells and platelets, and treatment of bone marrow deficiency
22. Improves lymphocyte count
23. Activates anti-inflammatory enzymes
24. Supports healthy liver function
25. Treats menopausal symptoms

26. Prevents morning sickness in the first trimester of pregnancy
27. Improves fertility
28. Strengthens muscles and bones
29. Supports normal kidney function
30. Improves memory and recall ability
31. Helps chronic dry cough
32. Alleviates anxiety and stress
33. Promotes cheerfulness and brightens the spirit
34. Improves weakened digestion

FreeLife Himalayan Goji is stated by Dr Earl Mindell and others that "Goji is Energy – Goji is earth's best battery. It stores energy. Energy = Life. Goji is the highest level of energy known. Dr Rick Honsell, Dr Earl Mendell's analyst and partner examined Goji against other Juces and here are his findings. Energy is measured on 2 scales: Bovis Energy Ratings and the Hertz Measurement. This is only a partial list but gives an example of how different products can be.

Bovis Energy Ratings and Hertz Measurement

Bovis Energy Ratings	Hertz Measurement
Noni....................17,000	Noni................. 0-
Sea Silver.......24.000	500 Sea Silver.......2,000
Limu Plus........54,000	Limu Plus..........2,000
Xango.............53,000	Xango...............2,300
GoJi...............355,000	GoJi..................6,000

Bovis Energy Ratings

Thanks to a French researcher in the 1930's by the name of Antoinne Bovis, we have a means to measure the "life force" or "natural earth energy" present in water, plants, rock formations and the like.

Ranging from zero to infinity, those trained in the required intuitive methods can assign a "Bovis" value to whatever they measure. For example, human beings show a reading on the Bovis scale of 6,500. Scientific research has correlated the counterclockwise or left spin of atoms and molecules. A Bovis reading below 6,500 is neutral for human life (i.e. life-depleting), and anything registering above 6,500 is essentially energy invigorating or enhancing to us. So, a clockwise or right spin correlates with a reading above 6,500 (i.e. life-enhancing). Besides mismanagement of the environment, readings below 6,500 are the effect of underground streams, geological faults, and Earth's magnetic grids. Several of Earth's energy vortices exceed 2,000,000 Bovis. FreeLife International's "Himalayan Goji Juice" shows a reading of 355,000 ... the highest reading that many health professionals have reported ever receiving.

The Hertz Energy Scale

Another energy unit... named for the German physicist Heinrich Rudolf Hertz (1857-1894), who proved in 1887 that energy is transmitted through a vacuum by electromagnetic waves.

In a world where science is recognizing "energy medicine" more and more and it's crucial role in releasing healing properties, these stats are a powerful confirmation of FreeLife's Himalayan Goji Juice playing an integral part (of the whole:-) in providing cutting-edge wellness products.

I have just mentioned that left spin is life depleting and right spin is life enhancing. Goji is the only juice among the juices mentioned that is right spin and can be used for life enhancing benefits. There is also value to juices that are left spin as left spin is used for detoxifying the body. Both are important.

As in foods that are left spin and right spin, Bruce Lipton explains that Particles come in pairs of spins. One is spinning left and one is spinning right. If one spin changes the other one changes its spin instantly to compliment it. More of Bruce Lipton on pg 179.

I usually look to products that are offered through network marketing. This way I am able to see the research and testing that has been done.

There is a benefit to rotating foods besides the boredom issue. I could do a chapter on that but you can do your own research. Just believe that a variety proves to have its' positives.

54

Minerals: Minerals, including trace minerals are necessary in every body function and are present in every human cell. Although the amount needed may be only a trace, problems may occur if we go without. We are continually encouraged to take our vitamins. We do not hear much of minerals and yet vitamins can not do their job without the use of minerals nor will the minerals work without the vitamins. They work together synergistically. Not only is our food stripped of the vitamin and mineral content by processing but the actual soil the food is grown on is depleted. Since this is the case it is extremely important to supplement our food intake with a good source of balanced minerals. All enzyme activities involve minerals whose function as coenzymes is enabling the body to perform all its functions, including energy production, growth and healing. Minerals are needed for the proper composition of all body fluids;: the formation of blood and bone, the maintenance of healthy nerve function, and the regulation of muscle tone, including muscles of the heart and cardiovascular system, arteries, veins, and capillaries. The best and probably the only way to get a perfect balance is to look to nature. All the trace minerals as well as the major minerals should be present and the minerals must have assimilability. Individual minerals are often given value on their own merit but the truth is that no single mineral can function without the others since they are synergistically related. There is evidence that minerals are conductors of the electrical currents in the body and provide a charge of positive or negative electrical molecules. Sea water is probably the best source of minerals. Sea water has the same chemical balance as the human blood. In fact in the case of an emergency, a doctor will use sea water in a transfusion if there is no blood available. There are some great sources of balanced minerals.

Food State has proven to have the key to a near perfect food matrix. A judge in California has ruled that Food State has the right to tell the truth. Food State can claim benefits.

Primal Cell Technologies, a 2007 company uses technologies that Nobel Prize winners have discovered in the last decade. The book "Molecules of Emotions" by Candace Pert tells the story of the 1999 Nobel Prize revealing a great discovery that can change all of the conditions of the body the world over including cancer, cardio, weight, allergies, diabetes, arthritis, prenatal among others. Candace

Pert has another book out entitled " Everything You Need to Feel Good or to Feel God" Can the right food do this for us? Some people think so.

Oxygen: I remember reading a book written by a man who had been nominated for a Nobel Prize for discovering that "Cancer can not live in an oxygenated system." What does it take to oxygenate a system? Water is the medium that carries the oxygen throughout the system. If you do not drink enough pure water, which has oxygen in it, it will not get to the cells. Some good sources for excellent oxygenation are the Chi Machine (for exercise) and Global Health Trax.

Water: I covered how to get good water in a previous section. Here I am explaining why it is so important, almost urgent, to use good water. Just a question and a note: Have you ever drunk ample water and discovered that you are still very thirsty and you are still dehydrated? One reason is because inferior water is often rejected in part by the cells. I have seen scientific pictures of healthy water and unhealthy water. There may be other requirements for the cells to accept the water such as good mineral content in the blood but that is another subject. Simply put, be good to your body and your body will be good to you.

Also if the minerals are taken out of the water you are drinking it is extremely important that you get your minerals from a different source. When you drink water that is not pure, you are drinking in pollutants that sometimes can not be eliminated out of the system. As I stated before, there are a number of ways to get pure water. Some are better than others. I prefer the whole home system and Bon Aqua is my choice. If you are renting, it is a good idea to get one of the other great systems around. If you are storing water in plastic containers, it is important to rotate the water as plastic can leach toxins into the water and affect the water in a harmful way. You used to be able to check the bottom of the container for a number that would indicate the least amount of leaching. Not so any more. Do not store water for long periods of time in plastic; and Rotate.

"GO RAW"?

Even though most people will not eat an entirely raw diet, I think most people can increase raw in their daily intake. What you put into your body is important. We need a quick pick up when we are in a hurry and crave things, and so we sometimes don't pay too much attention to what is best for us. Do raw when you can and do not worry about the rest. We just need to access help from the different ways we have available to us to make us feel better.

I want to introduce to you an idea that really is taking off and becoming more popular. Though this is one that I have not fully implemented into my own life, it is fascinating and there is something to it. We know that cooking and preservatives alter food so it takes out much of the benefit. If going raw is not your cup of tea, try the sprout and juicer part of it. You can also try the new discovery. **Primal Cell Technology**. This makes what you eat, good for you.

The report within this book speaks toward the value of going raw. It also contains in depth information about sugar. Do what you like with the information. It is not here to scare you. It is here to inform you because there *is* a way and it is really easy when you choose the things you like. No need to do it all. Have fun with it. When you feel well it is easier to eat well, so take a step at a time or go whole hog. Go with Goji if you want to stop the sugar craving and/or make it easier to eat raw and get healthy. It's up to you. Even if you Go Raw, it is believed to be impossible to get enough fiber.

FIBER: Betty Kamen PH.Ds' book on fiber is the best I've read. On the cover of her book "New Facts About FIBER" she says: "This book is for you if you are concerned about:

Weight control	Breast cancer Colon cancer
Prostate problems	Cholesterol levels Diabetes
Stomach disorders	Constipation Hemorrhoids
Diverticulitis	Hiatus hernia Heart disease
Ulcers	Longevity"

The benefits of Fiber is one of my favorite subjects because although there is no nutritional value, without it your body could not eliminate. There are many different fibers. A different fiber comes from different food. This is another example of variety being important. Although there are many fibers, they fall into two categories: Soluble and insoluble.

Soluble fiber
- Lowers cholesterol
- Reduces heart disease risk
- Improves blood sugar
- Lowers blood pressure
- Promotes growth of friendly flora

Insoluble fiber:
- Aids digestion
- Aids elimination
- Promotes regularity
- Contributes to bowel cleansing: This type of cleansing is like opening a plug. Your pipes (intestinal walls) are still in trouble without soluble fiber.

The more soluble the fiber, the more easily it is broken down, and therefore the nutrients in its complex structure are more usable. This quality differs significantly with the fiber source. Example: wheat bran is not as freely degraded as peas, carrots, cabbage, or apples.

When the fecal matter is broken up, it can be expelled. When the walls of your intestines are free from the impacted fecal matter, the nutrients can be absorbed and can be utilized.

Many people eat much more than they would need if the lining of the intestines were able to absorb the nutrients. Impacted intestines create a sense of need for more food than we really require to sustain us. Much of the food we feel driven to eat, cakes up inside us and adds to the antiques that are already there.

ENIVA
Want more energy?

How can Nanotechnology from the 1991 Nobel Prize winning Research and Research from both of the 2003 Nobel Prize Winners (Chemistry & Medicine) benefit your Health & Nutrition?

Why is 61% of the population overweight?
We have more food than any country - we eat but we are still hungry, right? Why?

Our body systems are starving for missing nutrients! – Our cells are malnourished.

Studies show our Foods & Vegetables have 2/3 fewer nutrients than 40 years ago.

Spinach has 45% less vitamin C **than 40 years ago**
Beets have 50 % less Vitamin C; Corn has 33% less Calcium
Apples have 41% less Vitamin A Greens have 85% less magnesium
Pineapples have 57% less Vitamin C

37% of the Population is deficient in Vitamin C, 61% is deficient in Magnesium,
78% of women – deficient in Calcium, 85% of total Population
50 % of Elderly Americans, deficient in Vitamin B 12, have Anemia

These deficiencies contribute to why:
> 61% of our population gets Diabetes
> 40% are projected to die of Stroke or Heart Attack
> 1/3 are projected to get Cancer
> 22% are projected tol get Alzheimer's, Dementia
> 60% have Arthritis
> 40% have Chronic Fatigue; most people may have multiple symptoms

It's created because of our lifestyle:
Lots of relentless Stress from Toxins, Free Radicals, Pollution, & Chemicals

Lots of Pollution & Toxins: Air, Food & Water
Not enough time for good diet, wrong food combinations and lack of exercise

Do you take supplements occasionally?
50% of the population does – **We Need Supplements, with the right isotopes.**

Most supplements are **Isolates**! Like –Ascorbic Acid for Vitamin C
Usually in tablet form – when in stomach it takes an hour or more to digest if at all.
If you place it in vinegar, heat on stove to 99 degrees – 45 min to hours to digest
Some of the pills go right thru you –(Salt Lake City Sewer –1,500 lbs per mo.)
Eniva Nutrition is:
Water Transported - Liquid based, Ionic Vitamins, Minerals, & Phytonutrients
Water base is nano, angstrom size; Nutrients are nano, angstrom size
(An angstrom is 1/10,000's of a micron) (Most bacteria are the size of a Micron)
The Water Carrier has a *negative charge* – toxic cells have a positive charge
Eniva bipasses the stomach – A *Study* shows Eniva enters the cells in 60 seconds-100% of the time.

Vibe is a comprehensive, all-in-one, anti-aging supplement that has 10 different technologies in sufficient quantity, balance and ratio: (2005 Physician Desk Ref.)
1. **Highest ORAC (Oxygen Radical Absorbance Capacity) rating. 83,000**
2. **Specialized Nano Water Technology (10-12 molecules/cluster down to 6-8 molecules per cluster – purified to USP23 standards.**
3. **Proprietary Vibrational Frequency Techniques.**
4. **Trade Protected Mineral/Nutrient Ionization Formula, Nano size**
5. **Human Matrix nutrient ratios that replicate natural ratios in the body.**

6. A specialized blend of anti-aging Components and DNA repair.
7. Bioactivation Technology to enhance digestion systems.
8. Heart Formula for reducing homocystein and supporting heart function.
9. 2003 Nobel Prize for Chemistry Technology for enhanced usage by the water channels in the cells. How to enhance Cell Hydration.
10. 2003 Nobel Prize in Chemistry Technology for enhanced usage by the calcium channels in the cells. This makes the sodium-potassium pump in the cells work better, creating ATP for energy of the cells in the body.

Vibe is equivalent to specific nutrients found in 13 tomatoes, 10 cups of raw green beans, 20 peaches, 35 cherries, 15 raw mangoes, 25 fresh walleye fillets, 5 beef steaks, 13 cracked wheat bread slices, 2.5 cups green tea, 10 percent Aloe Vera, plus hundreds of healthy nutrients from whole-food sources.

Vibe is vegetarian friendly!

How do the nutrients get into the Cells? The 2003 Nobel Prize in Chemistry by Peter Agre, M.D. for his discovery of **how nutrients "transport the cell membranes facilitated by water molecules and how the water channels are regulated."**
There are "water channels" through which nutrients are guided with the water molecules. There is a discovered protein, called Aquaporin that opens and closes the water channel to nutrients. **Water needs to be nano size** (usually angstrom size), and the Nobel Prize Research states that the **"water molecules need to have a negative charge to go into the cells."** "Thousands of millions of water molecules per second pass through one single water channel." "When the cells were placed in a water solution, those that had the protein in their membranes absorbed water by osmosis and swelled up while those that lacked the protein were not affected at all." "The membrane is not allowed to leak protons (+) of the water." "This is crucial because the difference in proton concentration between the inside and the outside of the cell is the basis of the cellular energy-

storage system. Selective is a central property of the channel. Water molecules worm their way through the narrow channel by orienting themselves in the local electrical field formed by the atoms of the channel wall. Protons (or rather oxonium ions, H20+) are stopped on the way and **rejected because of their positive charges."** "The water channels play a major part in the kidneys." "People with a deficiency of this hormone (vasopressin) are affected by the disease diabetes insipidly with a daily urine output of 10-15 litres." You can possibly postulate how beneficial it might be to have nano water and have it charged negatively.

How important is the electrical charge of the water to the Cells"
"Water molecules pass the channel single-file at a billionth of a second." Also, there are the "Ion channels" through which the sodium potassium mechanism creates energy. (Discussed in a latter part of this paper.)

How important is cell-to-cell communication with body systems? **What do we learn from the 1991 Nobel Prize?** (Erwin Neher & Bert Sakmann):
The key to the health of the cells has to do with the "ionic (charged atoms) of nutrition, "through which the cell communicates with its surroundings." In order to get into the cells from the receptors; there is an electrical potential difference between the inside and outside of the cell of 0.03 to 0.1 volts." **"The regulation of ion channels influences the life of the cell and its functions."** "This mechanism of new knowledge during the past 10 years has revolutionized modern biology, facilitated research, and contributed to the understanding of the cellular mechanisms underlying several diseases, including diabetes, epilepsy, cardio-vascular diseases, neuro-muscular disorders, and cystic fibrosis." "When a single ion channel opens, ions will move through the channel as an electric current, since they are charged." "ATP acts directly on a particular type of ion channel which controls the electric membrane potential of the cell."

1. The nutrient must have an ionic charge, hopefully a high one.
2. The ionic charged nutrient potential of every vitamin, mineral, phytonutrient must be higher on the outside of the cell than on the inside to travel through the ion

channel in each cell's membrane to provide enough energy to the cell.
3. It needs to be angstrom size to go into the cell.
4. It has to be transported with water & protein (1996 Nobel Prize research)
5. The Nutrient Receptor (1 Million receptors on each cell) has to recognize the nutrient (the electromagnetic signal). (1996 Nobel Prize)

How do you take care of free-radicals in your body? **VIBE has the highest ORAC** (Oxygen Radical Absorbance Capacity) score of any product:

Sea Silver	2,880	**Tahitian Noni**	5,280
Goji	12,160	**Xango**	16,960
Berry Young Juice	32,000	**Enive VIBE**	**83,200**

How do you take care of DNA repair in your body?
Research shows our cells die after reproducing 60-80 times. After that the Telomeres (ends of the DNA strands which regulate cell division) shorten and can no longer allow the cell to divide. 1/3 or more of the damaged DNA needs repair. How can you correct this? (see the book, EXCITOTOXINS, Russell L. Blaylock, M.D.)
Vibe (a vibrational energy, mineral product) uses D-Ribose and other co factors which increases ATP for energy and endurance, supporting Muscle Recovery and causing a synthesis of neculeotides for DNA repair. Enzymes, nutrition, & amino acids along with D-Ribose is important for DNA repair.

How to reduce the risk for Heart Attack, Stroke, Diabetes, Cancer, & Alzheimer's?
"Doctor James Braly M.D. (Life Stream Recovery-Laguna Hills, CA.) & Patrick Holford (Institute for Optimum Nutrition) found 70% of the population has a High Homecystein above 9. Also, a 1992 Study of 14,000 Male M.D.'s found they have a 3 times greater risk of having a heart-attack – (Newsweek)

"Dr. Braly found lowered Homocystein in the body will:
   "Reduce the Risk of Heart Attack by 80%"
   "Risk of Strokes by 82%"   "Risk of Diabetes by 90%"
   "Risk of Cancer by 33%"   "Risk of Alzheimer's by 50%"

"Dr. Braly found the following nutrients lower Homostyeine:
Folic Acid, Vitamin A, C, E, Selenium, CoQ10, L-Carnitine, Malic Acid, B , B 12 & Lecithin. These nutrients in Vibe's Heart Complex is designed to lower Homocysteine. Also, JAMA 1997; 277 (22): 1775-1781, a Study of 800 heart patients."

VIBE is listed in the Physicians' Desk Reference- Doctors can prescribe it.

1991 Nobel Prize in Physiology or Medicine-Erwin Neher * Bert Sakmann , "For new discoveries concerning the function of ion channels in cells"

1991 Nobel Prize Summary:
"Each living cell is surrounded by a membrane which separates the world within the cell from its exterior. In this membrane there are channels (controlled by the receptors), through which the cell communicates with its surroundings. These channels consist of single molecules or complexes of molecules and have the ability to allow passage of charged atoms, that is ions. The regulation of ion channels influences the life of the cell and its function under normal and pathological conditions. The Nobel Prize in Medicine is awarded for the discovery of the function of ion channels... They have demonstrated what happens during the opening or closure of an ion channel with a receptor localized to one part of the channel molecule which upon activation alters its shape. They show parts of the molecule that constitute the sensor and the interior wall of the channel. They also showed how the channel regulates the passage of positively or negatively charged ions."

"This new knowledge and this new analytical tool has during the past 10 years revolutionized modern biology, facilitated research, and contributed to the understanding of the cellular mechanisms underlying several diseases, including diabetes, cystic fibrosis, epilepsy, cardio-vascular diseases, and neuro-muscular disorders."

What happens Inside the Cell?
"Inside the cell differs from its outside. There is a difference in electrical potential, amounting to 0.03 to 0.1 volts, known as the membrane potential. The cell uses the membrane potential in

64

several ways. By rapidly opening channels for sodium ions the membrane potential is altered radically within a thousandth of a second. Cells in the nervous system communicate with each other by means of electrical signals of around a tenth of a volt that rapidly travel along the nerve processes. When they reach the point of contact between 2 cells – the synapse either induces the release of a transmitter substance or a closure of the ion channel. This substance affects receptors on the target cell, often by opening ion channels. The membrane potential is hereby altered so that the cell is stimulated or inhibited. The nervous system consists of a series of networks each comprised of nerve cells connected by synapses with different functions. New memory traces in the brain are for example created by altering the number of available ion channels in the synapses of a given network."

What happens outside the cell?
"Fluids outside the cells within the body ideally have a pH of 7.4.-7.5 (above 7.0 is alkaline)(if your are well). This fluid enters the cell, is depleted and exits the cell having a pH of 6.8. The action of fluids going in and out of the cells at these levels create an electrical charge of 70 milivolts. If the body cannot create this electrical charge on the outside of the cell, it becomes essential to life for nutrients to be converted into electricity. Absent this charge, and the cells cannot communicate. This charge is reliant on a trigger mechanism composed of the right nutrients. If these nutrients are lacking, the body must use its own stored-up supply of Calcium in the bones. As the level of minerals goes down, oxygen supply decreases and the body becomes susceptible to diseases, including all cancers. Over 75 years ago, Otto Warburg was awarded two Nobel prizes—for his theories that cancer is caused by weakened cell respiration due to lack of oxygen at the cell level. According to Warburg, damaged cell respiration causes fermentation, resulting in acidity at the cellular level. Dr. Warburg in his Nobel Prize winning paper, illustrated that the environment of the cancer cell is everything. A cell undergoes an adverse change in that it no longer takes in oxygen to convert glucose into energy. In the absence of oxygen the cell reverts to a survival nutrition program to nourish itself by converting glucose to cell division through the process of fermentation. The lactic acid produced by fermentation lowers the cell pH--(the acid/alkaline balance) and destroys the ability of DNA

and RNA to control cell division allowing the cancer cells then to begin multiplying. The lactic acid simultaneously causes severe lose that destroy cell enzymes and the cancer appears as a rapidly growing external cell covering the core of dead cells. Research by Keith Brewer, PhD and H.E. Satori has shown that raising the pH or oxygen content, range of a cell to pH 8.0 creates a death environment for cancer.

Despite the public taking Calcium, studies show 80% of the population is deficient because only about 5% is usable by the body from most products. These deficiencies contribute to over 150 diseases. Scientist instruct that for calcium to be bio-available, the formulation must have the correct ration of Calcium and its elemental partner **Magnesium that must have its trigger Vitamin D plus vitamin A and then must be ionized. It must be in a liquid form so as not to plug up the arteries and veins.**

"All cells function in a similar way. Life itself begins with a change in membrane potential. As the sperm merges with the egg cell at the instant of fertilization ion channels are activated. The resultant change in membrane potential prevents the access of other sperm cells. All cells - nerve cells, gland cells, and blood cells – have a characteristic set of ion channels that enable them to carry out their specific functions. The ion channels consist of single molecules or complexes of molecules, which form the wall of the channel that traverses the cell membrane and connects the exterior to the interior of the cell. The diameter of the channel is so small that it corresponds to that of a single ion (0.5-0.6 millionths of a millimeter) An immediate change in the shape of the molecule leads to either an opening or a closure of the ion channel. This can occur upon activation of the receptor part of the molecule that leads to either an opening or a closure of the ion channel..."

How does an Ion Channel Operate?
"When a single ion channel opens, ions will move through the channel as an electric current, since they are charged. Some are positively charged, while others are negatively charged. Sometimes, there are 2 rings of positively or negatively charged amino acids that form an ionic filter which permit ions with an opposite charge to pass through the filter (of the cell membrane). Neher and Sakman's

66

scientific achievements have radically changed our view on the function of the cell and the contents of text books on cell biology..."

Regulation of Ion Channel Function:
"Also, the basal mechanism underlying the secretion of insulin have been identified. The level of blood glucose controls the level of glucose within the insulin-forming cell, which in turn regulates the level of the energy rich substance **ATP**. **ATP** acts directly on a particular type of ion channel which controls the electric membrane potential of the cell. The change of membrane potential then indirectly influences other ion channels, which permit calcium ions to pass into the cell. The calcium ions subsequently trigger the insulin secretion. In diabetes, the insulin secretion is out of order. Certain drugs commonly used to stimulate insulin secretions in diabetes act directly on the ATP channels..."

References:
Alberts et al: The Molecular Biology of the Cell, Garland Press, 1990 pp. 156, 312-326
Grillner, S.I.; Calder, N. Scientic Europ. Foundation Scientific Europe, 1990
Grillner, S. & Hokfelt, t.: Svindlande snabb utveckling pragler neurovetenskapen. Lakartidiningen 1990, 87, 27777-27786.
Rosman, P. & Fredholm, B.B.: Jonkanaler – molekylar bakgrund till nervtransmission. Lakartidningen 1991, 88, 2868-2877.

How important is the Sodium Potassium Pump concept to creating Energy (ATP)?
New Research (2003 Nobel Prize) shows how important ion mechanisms are to the health of individual cells, particularly for the creation of energy (ATP) in the Sodium-Potassium Pump of the cell. It requires Calcium, Magnesium, Sodium, and Potassium in the right highly ionic state, with the right isotopes for each mineral aligned and have the right spin, and in the right combination of each mineral to have a positive synergistic effect with each ingredient. In addition to the right isotopes in the mix, there must be also:
1. Protein, Vitamin D., Iron (Isotope 57), Manganese (Isotope 28), Zinc (Isotope 72), and mostly Magnesium (Isotope 28), all in a high ionic state with isotope 46 (Calcium).

Manganese needs to have Zinc, Vitamin E, B1, Vitamin C, and Vitamin K **in order for Calcium to process correctly**.

2. Vitamin D and Magnesium (Isotope 28) are needed **to make Sodium.**
3. Calcium (Isotope 46), and Magnesium (Isotope 28) are needed in order **to make Potassium.**
4. Calcium, Phosphorus (Isotope 34), Zinc, Vitamin B 1, Vitamin B 6, Vitamin C, and Vitamin D need to work in a high ionic state **to make Magnesium.**

All of these in the right combinations appear to be in Vibe. Just taking a Calcium-Magnesium pill, a potassium pill, or any other combination of supplements won't give you higher energy if you have the wrong form or wrong isotope number.

What happens if you have the wrong kind of Calcium, Potassium, & Sodium Magnesium? These minerals need to be in a liquid, ionic state, not pill form to allow the electric ions to form together when water breaks the ionic bonds, the positive ions and negative ions multiply when you add water which breaks the ionic bonds and allows the energy of the nutrients to increase. Also, most Calcium manufacturers use Calcium 40 Isotope, when you have our Calcium of 46 Isotopes in the Sodium Potassium Pump, which creates ATP energy it works synergistically with Potassium at a Maximum potential. The Isotopes determine the spin of the molecules, which is key to increasing energy (right spin) or detoxing the cell (left spin).

MD's warn that getting too much Calcium supplementation or the wrong kind of Calcium can be deposited in the joints, in the muscles, and clog the arteries, lymph, veins, and blood vessels.

1. **How does the Sodium-Potassium Pump create energy in our cells? And; How do the Voltage Membrane Channels open & close and the Calcium Cell Channels work? NEW RESEARCH-2003 NOBEL PRIZE – Dr Roderick MacKinnon tells us how.**

"Voltage dependent ion channels bring an explosive, and then restorative burst of energy to the otherwise placid cell membrane.

In a nerve cell, for example, the explosive burst of the neurotransmitter, glutamate, hits a sensitive receptor on the cell's surface for a sea of change. Glutamate triggers sodium-conducting channels on the cell's surface to open up and allow positively charged sodium to flow into the negatively charged interior of the cell instantly, neighboring voltage dependent sodium channels (NAV) open in response for more sodium to enter, creating an upset in the normal negative inside, positive outside voltage common to all living cells. As soon as the explosive cascade of sodium channeling begins, hyper-sensitive voltage dependent potassium channels (Kv) along the same cell's surface sense the catastrophic switching of the charge value inside the cell and in their own domino effect, open up to allow positive charged ions to quickly flow out of the cell. This movement restores a cell's normal negative inside and positive outside charge value. The cell returns to its former calm. The entire sequence of events takes only a few milliseconds, and occurs tens of thousands of times every day in human beings. Without this hair-trigger electric system life would be more than calm. There would be scant possibility of thinking, breathing, or movement. Ion channels opened or closed positions have an impact on the charged value of the cell membrane."

2. **How does Magnesium increase the Cellular Membrane Potential? "Magnesium is the most important binder of minerals in the body for the creation of ATP that gives us energy."** Magnesium:
   a. "Influences the metabolic reactions for the use and supply of energy.
   b. "Neutralizes the negative charges on the outside of cells increasing the electrolyte balance inside and outside the cell causing the body to create **more ATP for energy**.
   c. "The magnesium ion is larger, in its hydrate state, than the Calcium ion displacing calcium in the calcium channel. Its effect causes:
      1. " The blood vessels to dilate."
      2. "The oxygen balance of the cells to improve, increase supply and lower oxygen consumption."
      3. " The inhibition of Magnesium causes the release of Neurotransmitters; Adrenaline and Non

adrenaline for reducing risk of heart disease and reduced stress."
4. "It feeds the nerves and the Autonomic Nervous System."
5. "It is one of the main ingredient for the creation of ATP energy."

Magnesium works on: Headaches, dislocations, confusion, poor concentration, nervousness, jumpiness, migraine, cramps in the muscles of face, neck, shoulder, and entire vertebral column, palpitation, arrhythmia, gastrointestinal cramps, nausea, vomiting, diarrhea, urinary tract cramps, uterine cramps, tingling of the hands, numbness, constipation, thigh and calf cramps, cramps and tingling in the soles of the feet and toes.

3. **How do you increase the electrical energy potential by putting the product in a small amount of water?**
Professor Hoff, Bio Chemist, Dept. of Energy says, "ionic bonds do not conduct electricity. However, when a compound dissolves in water, the inter-ion bonds are broken. This enables the + and – ions to move about in the Solution. These positive and negative ions gather together to create electricity in the body increasing the energy." This is the high ionic charge you see on the ionic meter. Vibe is the highest we have found.

4. **How do you increase enzyme activity in the body?** Dr. Kuhn, a Scientist at the Lewis Center, says, "The activity of enzymes depends on the ionic conditions (of the substrate) and the pH of the surroundings." **When a product has a high ionic nature there is a higher enzyme activity. Vibe is highly ionic.** The HRM water you drink has a high pH of around 8 and will increase the ionic state.

BIOENERGETIC – "GIBBS FREE ENERGY"

How can you increase metabolism (to increase the energy of ATP) in the cell?
1. **"Metabolism is the sum of all chemical reactions."**
2. **"Metabolism involves– catabolism (left spin products) and/or anabolism (right spin products)" "Catabolism (left spin products) and Anabolism (right spin**

70

products) are energy coupled in order to release energy."

3. "Catabolism (left spin products) decreases free energy, possesses less stored energy than do the reactants." "It must give off (lose) some free energy as it goes forward.." "This results in less free energy being produced from the product itself."

4. "Anabolic (right hand spin products) posses more energy than do the reactants." "Requires a net input of free energy to proceed." "This results in more free energy than what is acquired from the products

5. "The rate at which the reaction (ATP) goes forward depends on the activation energy necessary to initiate the reaction."

6. "Energy must be supplied to drive the reaction forward."

In order to make everything work to maximum benefit, you need the cofactors of B Vitamins.

REFERENCES

Professor Hoff, Bio Chemist, Dept. of Energy

2003 Nobel Prize (Medicine) – Dr. Roderick MacKinnon

2003 Nobel Prize (Chemistry) - Peter Agre, M.D

1991 Nobel Prize (Medicine) cell-to-cell communication Erwin Neher & Bert Sakmann

Alberts et al: The Molecular Biology of the Cell, Garland Press, 1990 pp. 156, 312-326

Grillner, S.I.; Calder, N. Scientic Europe. Foundation Scientific Europe, 1990

Grillner, S. & Hokfelt, t.: Svindlande snabb utveckling pragler neurovetenskapen. Lakartidiningen 1990, 87, 27777-27786.

Newsweek, Aug. 11, 1997; Farmingham Heart Study (1995); NEJM 1995; 332(5)286-91

Rosman, P. & Fredholm, B.B.: Jonkanaler – molekylar bakgrund till nervtransmission. Lakartidningen 1991, 88, 2868-2877.

PRIMAL CELL TECHNOLOGIES

With all the recent research of scientists we know, we are learning new ways and new technologies to give us health and wellness. This adds to our wisdom and can help us make smart choices.

When food is altered or processed, it is not complete. There are 12 tests that food can go through to show the highest level of benefit. There are good ones and not so good ones. Do any of them pass all requirements to claim ultimate benefits? PRIMAL CELL TECHNOLOGIES does. It makes the foods you eat, good for you.

1) IONIC: The body is electric. If the product you put in your body is not electric. It is not complete. We need to be electric.
2) OBSORBSION: We are a large percent water. Some say 70% others say 90%. If the product does not absorb in water the body can not use it effectively.
3) ENERGY: Since we are made up of energy, having the product that has the energy spin in the proper way is essential.
4) PLATEAU for ENERGY: The energy that has high frequency provides more peaceful feeling and less stress.
5) UTILIZATION: The higher the percentage, the better. Some really good products have a fairly low utilization or assimilation.
6) ENERGY BALANCE: Your body's energy should be balanced. There are times when a temporary imbalance can work for an isolated incident for speedy recovery on a location. It will weaken other areas but it should be O.K. for short term use.
7) BIO MERIDIAN. The 12 meridians should be an average of 50%, since each meridian shares energy with another meridian, if one is higher, the other one would be lower. It needs to be in proper balance.
8) MEASURE THE EFFECT ON THE QUANTUM FIELD: We are finding the Quantum Field has a major bearing on our health.
9) COMPARISON. Comparison with other products
10) BLOOD TYPE: There are some ingredients that work well with all Blood Types. If not, the product can work on one blood type and not on another.
11) METABOLIC TYPE: work with hormones and neuro-peptides
12) SYNERGISTIC EFFECTS: How do all the parts work together?

THE MISSING LINK
Technology in the discovery
We are all made up of energy. Pretty much everything is made up of energy. If the energy we are made up of is fragmented, absolute mental and physical health is not obtained.

Layers of Light

Layers of Light International, Inc. is dedicated "To Promoting Peace and Transforming Humanity by Empowering Individuals to Achieve Higher Consciousness and Sustained Wellness

Our M-Power Life System immediately enhances the Five Factors of physical performance including: balance, coordination, flexibility, strength and endurance while supporting the energy signals in the brain responsible for achieving higher levels of consciousness, mental clarity, calmness, focus and recall.

Sari Y. Suttka, D.C. has spent over 20 years researching combined sciences in the health field including formulating and testing products to support this vision. Simply stated, your highest potential and sustained wellness revolves around being aligned in Mind, Body and Spirit, in other words: the alignment of your Primary Energy Field to the Quantum Field.

In the last few decades, over half of all inventions have been quantum based. Leading experts in this field such as David Bohm Ph.D., Karl Pribram Ph.D., Stewart Hammeroff M.D., Roger Penrose Ph.D., Harold Puthoff Ph.D., V. Vernon Woolf Ph.D. and Ronald Jones Ph.D. have contributed an advanced and respectful body of work that identifies man as a multi-dimensional being with a consciousness that is connective and collective.

The paradigm of modern medicine ignores these findings and continues to separate body and spirit. The ancient cultures including Native Americans, China, Tibet, India, Egypt, etc. identify the quantum field in the assessment of wellness, but either ignores or was unaware of the impact of the technology of man's genius and artificial intelligence of the Third Millennium.

73

Such technologies include electro-pollution (cell phones, computers, televisions, radios, etc.) including fluorescent lighting, and chemical pollution (over 80,000 manmade chemicals in our vital life space of air, food and water), including toxic vapors and synthetic pharmaceuticals. These man-made "advancements" of technology, while enhancing our lifestyle, are creating energy interrupters that have a significant detrimental effect on each of us. For additional information refer to www.ewg.org.

It is the belief of Layers of Light International, Inc. that to empower lives we must acknowledge our responsibility to our ourselves, each other and to the Planet Biosphere with regard to wellness and the interruptions that prevent us from achieving our full energy potential. With this understanding, a new paradigm of wellness must be created to respect the holistic knowledge of who we are in our current position in the Biosphere and at the same time identify the interruptions that prevent us from achieving our full energy potential. Thus, were born the Fusion Formulas™: Quantum Life Support for the 21st Century™.

> Our Mission is: "To Promote Peace and Transform Humanity by Empowering Individuals to Achieve Higher Consciousness and Sustained Wellness."
>
> Layers of Light International, Inc is the first company to provide products that organize quantum energy to achieve Peace, Love and Wellness in the biosphere.
>
> When using the Fusion Formulas™, you will immediately **experience increased strength, flexibility, balance, coordination and endurance.**

The M-Power™ Life System elevates the energy of the body to allow alignment with the Primary Energy Source and empowers individuals to achieve higher consciousness and sustained wellness.

Research in modern Quantum Physics has led to the identification of man as a multidimensional, collective conscious being. **Fusion Formulas™** were created as a practical application that combines Newtonian Physics with Quantum theory. The layering of the

74

products, referred to as Quantum layer one through Quantum layer 5, attempts to organize this multi-dimensional aspect to achieve alignment of man's *Primary Energy Field.*

Fusion Formulas™ were created to provide synergistic coherence of energy from the inside-out and from the outside-in of the body. When one focuses on the inside-out, man's electrical nature and the optimum millivoltage at the cellular level must be appreciated. The goal is to achieve synchronization and balancing of brain signals to create coherence in the physical body with an aerobic capacity of eighty five percent (85%) at the cellular level, while enhancing the **five factors** of physical performance: **balance, coordination, flexibility, strength and endurance.**

The hierarchy of sustaining human life at optimum levels begins with oxygen, water, minerals, glucose, millivoltage, Ph (acid – alkaline), temperature, nucleic acids, amino acids, fatty acids, enzymes and vitamins. This "order" holds true in the emergency room and for maintaining optimum wellness. Two of the **Fusion Formulas™** , *Q-Power™ Water* and *Q-Power™ Spray* impact the Quantum nature of man by aligning the multidimensional layers of subtle energy. The "Fusion" of these two products supports higher consciousness while providing the primary and secondary requirements for "life support." *Q-Power™ Water* provides the highest concentration of stabilized oxygen found in water, which is then absorbed through the venous system by diffusion, bypassing the lungs.

Q-Power™ Marine Matrix is a 100% certified organic whole raw vegan food concentrate. It was primarily created to promote Peace within, which is the primary resonance of sustained wellness. This can be measured by salivary PH remaining alkaline in the presence of acidic foods. It is a naturally balanced electrolyte providing the proper ration of major minerals and rare earth trace minerals only found in the vegetation of the ocean. Inherent within the Matrix are potent nutritional factors and alkalizing properties naturally found in the electro magnetic energy of the sun and sea.

The outside-in **Fusion Formulas™**, Quantum layers: the *M-Power™ Pouch* and Quantum Matrix, the *Q-Power™ Spray* address the electro-pollution (EMF's), toxic vapors, scars, surgery, trauma, body piercing, tattoos etc. by organizing the Quantum subtle energies of which we are composed.

"Wellness is multidimensional. It is an accepted scientific fact that there are at least ten dimensions enfolded into physical reality. Traditionally science and health treatment modalities have been based upon a four-dimensional model of reality wherein we experience depth, width, height and the passage of time. With the unveiling of multiple dimensions of reality comes new understanding that everything is conscious, made of hyperspacial information spinners, quantum potential fields, holographic dynamics, quantum forces, Frohlich frequencies and parallel worlds. Those who serve the public trust for wellness must deal with these dimensions and how they influence personal reality and the wellness process." [1]

To this end **Fusion Formulas™** were created applying the concepts of theoretical physics and Quantum consciousness to "Promote Peace and Transform Humanity by Empowering Individuals to Achieve Higher Consciousness and Sustained Wellness"

"The Phenomena will Persist – although the Experience is Real"

[1] Victor Vernon Wolfe, Ph.D. "The Wellness Manifesto"

Quantum Life Support for the 21st Century
An inherent order to all life. If we could, take a moment and reflect on survival. Without oxygen how long could we survive? Without water how long could we survive? When we become ill and go to the hospital they administer a drip of saline to support hydration and electrolytes. Often they administer glucose as well. If we have a heart attack the defibrillator paddles are used for an electrical jump-start.

Modern medicine approaches life-support in a specific order: oxygen, water (hydration), minerals (electrolytes), glucose (fuel), etc. When symptoms of a lesser urgency arise the focus is on drugs not oxygen, water or minerals. The order of life-support (survival) or sustained wellness remains the same; oxygen, water, minerals. If oxygen, water, minerals, glucose and millivoltage are compromised, the vitamins and amino acids you are taking in the form of food or supplements are not being assimilated or utilized sufficiently.

The order in which Fusion Formulas are recommended comply with Life Support for the 21 st Century. The air we breathe, the food we eat and the water we drink are all polluted with over 80,000 man-made chemicals. Therefore our quality of life and life-space have been compromised. We must align ourselves to a higher source of energy to achieve sustained wellness in the 21st century. The alignment, first and foremost is to our Primary Energy Field. This is achieved with the combined Fusion Formulas of Q-Power™ Water and Q-Power™ Spray. Our other M-Power™ Products are formulated to address the energy interrupters man has created.

The addition of recommended artist's music support the "space" in which we work, study, recuperate and play. The organizing harmonics of certain artists' music affect the brain signals enhancing a state of peace which promotes the mission of Layers of Light International, Inc. We proudly offer the compositions of Mark Romero, Peter Sterling and Gemma.

Listed below are details regarding the Quantum Field and Electrical Field

Quantum Field

1. **Primary Energy Alignment** - The success of the Mission depends upon maintaining our Primary Energy Alignment. It is tested with fingertips touching the crown of the head (top-center), and by Applied Kinesiology (AK), arm strength should hold strong. At this point, by pointing your fingertips to the feet, by Applied Kinesiology (AK), arm strength should be weak.

   A secondary energy or back up occurs in **polarization**. Initially, the crown (top of the head) and feet both test strong by Applied Kinesiology (AK). Over time, a reversal of energy causes the feet to be strong and the crown to test weak. Ultimately, both the crown and the feet will test weak.

The implication is energy exhaustion. This is referred to as *Manipulation of Energy*.

Only the ●Q-Power™ Water and ●Q-Power™ Spray when used together will hold your Primary Energy Alignment. This is referred to as *Harnessing Energy*.

2. **Electrical Brain** – The outside-in support for the brain is the ●M-Power™ Pouch and ●Q-Power™ Spray.●Q-Power™ Water and ●M-Power™ Matrix enhance and supercharge the signals.
3. **Electrical Body** – The M-Power™ System is required for the nullification of electrical interrupters.
4. **Mind** – ●●The number one priority is Primary Energy Alignment. Energy support from ◆M-Power™ Matrix, ● and the ●M-Power™ Pouch affect Harmonization and Coherence of Brain signals.

5-Factors and Gravity - ●●●A requirement of a Fusion Formula™ is that it must enhance balance, coordination, flexibility, strength, and endurance. Optimal Center of Gravity is a shift that occurs between the body's center of mass and the downward force of gravity.

Electrical Field

Oxygen:

●Q-Power™ **Water** supplies 64.8 mg of stabilized oxygen per liter of water. The use of this water has been shown to enhance through the portal vein of the liver at least 10% or more of oxygen. The liver's primary function is detoxification, and with the added uptake of oxygen into the liver, it makes this detoxification mechanism much more efficient. All toxins, chemicals and biologically harmful materials have to go through this detoxification process. Enormous amounts of harmful by-products come from harmful microbes in the gut.

Q-Power™ Spray - This affects the Quantum field nullifying Energy Interrupters (such as Deep Emotional Issues, Neurological Entrapments, etc.) as well as other Energy Interrupters (such a vapors, etc.) that compete with oxygen molecules that affect the physical environment.

Water:

Q-Power™ Water and Q-Power™ Spray carry the message of the Mission Inside-Out and Outside-In.

M-Power™ Pouch – This harnesses energy into the body, including containing energies that support the resonant frequency of water.

Minerals:

The M-Power™ Pouch provides a resonant frequency which organizes the minerals.

The Q-Power™ Water carries the energy message of the Mission, which further organizes the minerals.

Glucose:

Millivoltage: The voltage of a cell averages 70-90 mv. However, this average depends upon having the optimum content of oxygen, water, minerals and glucose. This is accomplished with Q-Power™ Water, M-Power™ Marine Matrix, M-Power™ Pouch and Q-Power™ Spray.

pH Acid-Alkaline: The Q-Power™ Water, M-Power™ Marine Matrix provide the support for physiologic pH balance to occur in the body.

Body Temperature: Water in general affects the thermostat of the body. The M-Power™ Marine

Matrix supports the hydration level of the body, thereby affecting temperature.

Nucleic Acids DNA/RNA: Water is responsible for the scaffolding, folding and unfolding of DNA. The support for the processing of information exchange is supplied by both the · Q-Power™ Water and ◆M-Power™ Marine Matrix.

Amino Acids:

▪Q-Power™ Marine Matrix is the major supplier of the Amino Acid building blocks of collagen. Formulated for processing of information through the connective tissues of the body.

▪M-Power™ Water carries the message of organization, while the ◆M-Power™ Marine Matrix supplies the co-factors necessary for energy metabolism.

Fatty Acids:

◆Q-Power™ Marine Matrix supports Fatty Acid metabolism.

◆Q-Power™ Water carries the message necessary for fatty acid energy metabolism.

Enzymes:

▪Q-Power™ Marine Matrix provides the minerals that act as catalysts or "starter" molecules for enzymes to do their work.

◆Q-Power™ Water and ˮ Q-Power™ Marine Matrix provide all aspects of enzyme function.

B-Vitamins:

⦁Q-Power™ Marine Matrix is the major supplier of organisms, which manufacture all the B-Vitamins necessary for energy metabolism.

⦁Q-Power™ Water contains the energy of the message of the Mission to sustain this activity of energy metabolism.

Product Question and Answer

If you would prefer a printable PDF version of our FAQs, please see web site www.2lolii.com/dandyone

1. What is the Product that Layers of Light International, Inc. is sharing with people?
2. Can I just use the M-Power™ Pouch, or is it necessary to use the other M-Power™ products?
3. What is the definition of quantum?
4. Why is Layering important?
5. What are energy interrupters?
6. Why do people get different results from the M-Power™ Pouch?
7. How do you define electrical and why is it important?
8. What kind of results can we expect from the water?
9. How are the M-Power™ energies put into the products?
10. How much M-Power™ Marine Matrix and M-Power™ Spray should I take in a day?
11. What is the difference between the Layers of Light recommended organizing music versus all other music?
12. Are there any side-effects from using these products?
13. What is the shelf life of our M-Power™ products?
14. What does M-Power™ stand for?
15. What is inside the M-Power™ Pouch?
16. Should I wear the M-Power™ Pouch all the time?
17. Is the M-Power™ Pouch washable? What if I get it wet?
18. Is the M-Power™ System a medical device and can it be used to cure disease?
19. There are many energy products on the market. What separates the M-Power™ Products from the others?

1. What is the Product that Layers of Light International, Inc. is introducing?

The core product is called the "M-Power™ Life System" and is composed of Fusion Formulas™. The M-Power™ Life System consists of three components, 1. Q-Power™ Marine Matrix 2. Q-Power™ Spray and 3. M-Power™ Pouch. Fusion Formulas™ not only enhance the five physical factors of performance. Additionally our products support higher consciousness for sustained wellness. Each additional M-Power™ product targets a specific layer of disorganization in our energy field.

2. Can I just use the M-Power™ Pouch, or is it necessary to use the other M-Power™ products?

This product was designed to be used within a system of the three components mentioned above. All information is organized in ranges of frequencies much like your radio. The M-Power™ Pouch organizes what we refer to a Quantum Layer 4 organization of frequencies. Our studies have shown that in order to use the M-Power™ Pouch successfully you must use the Q-Power™ Marine Matrix and the Q-Power™ Spray to make sure you are electrical and to utilize the increase in energy.

3. What is the definition of quantum? Quantum is the study of the space that exists between an atom and an electron as well as the space within an atom.

4. Why is Layering important?

Each Quantum Layer formula was designed to work synergistically to address different layers of vibration within the body. Collectively the fusion formulas™ presently address the multitude of energy interrupters that each of us are exposed to on a daily bases.

5. What are energy interrupters?

Things that disrupt our normal energy, such as: the exposure to toxic pollution from the 80,000 man-made chemicals that invade our life space of air, food and water, as well as Electro-Pollution, artificial
82

lighting, medications, scars, tattoos, body piercing, metals either worn or in our teeth and jewelry.

6. Why do people get different results from the M-Power™ Pouch?

The M-Power Pouch was never designed to be used alone; it is a component of the M-Power System to be used with the M-Power™ Marine Matrix and the Q-Power™ Spray. Additionally each individual's vibration is disorganized differently depending on their level of exposure to energy interrupters.

7. How do you define electrical and why is it important?

Each of the cells in your body has a specific electrical voltage. A healthy cell is between 70mv and 90mv. When the millivoltage of the cell drops down to around 15mv due to an energy interrupter the cell becomes, unhealthy and susceptible to diseases, like cancer. The Q-Power™ Marine Matrix was formulated to support the higher millivoltage of the cell.

8. What kind of results can we expect from the water?

The Q-Power™ Oxygenated Water addresses the immediate enhancement of physical performance of balance, coordination, strength, flexibility and endurance. Additionally, as is proven by brain maps we see a balance of signals in the brain which support enhanced focus and concentration. Extra Oxygen is provided to the liver to support the release of toxins. Drinking water every 15 minutes if you are in serious condition is important.

9. How are the M-Power™ energies put into the products?

This is a proprietary process.

10. How much Q-Power™ Marine Matrix should I take in a day?

Originally it was discovered that it was best to take when the tulleric current is highest. However it has been discovered that if you look up while taking the product it is equally optimal.

11. What is the difference between the Layers of Light recommended organizing music versus all other music?

We have found that some music has energy organizing frequencies and other music has energy disorganizing frequencies. Through our research with brain mapping we have identified music that is compatible with our M-Power™ system and our mission to achieve higher consciousness.

12. Are there any side-effects from using these products?

All of the ingredients in the M-Power™ products are natural and safe for human consumption, as well as external application. The M-Power™ system does assist in detoxifying the body so it is important to drink enough water to support this effort. To limit the side-effects of detoxification you must use the M-Power™ Marine Matrix when wearing the M-Power™ Pouch.

13. What is the shelf life of our M-Power™ products?

The M-Power™ Pouch contents are life long. The consumable M-Power™ Products have an expiration date on each label.

14. What does M-Power™ stand for?

The "M" stands for Mission Power which embodies the directive of the mission statement of Layers of Light International.

15. What is inside the M-Power™ Pouch?

The physical contents of the M-Power™ Pouch is a crystalline quartz matrix including amethyst. The crystalline matrix is designed to hold a coherent bio-energy field in the presence of disorganizing electro-magnetic-frequencies.

16. Should I wear the M-Power™ Pouch all the time?

Yes. The Pouch can be worn 24/7 and is designed to wear while you sleep. The proper placement of the Pouch is in the front of the body, between the neck and waist. If used elsewhere, it will be ineffective. It is very important to remember to take the M-Power™ Marine Matrix and M-Power™ Spray daily with water.

17. Is the M-Power™ Pouch washable? What if I get it wet?

Yes, it is washable. Please be gentle and wash by hand with mild liquid soap. Rinse and hang to dry. It is currently being used in wetsuits for surfing and diving. If the pouch gets wet, squeeze out extra water between a towel and hang to dry. Do not place in clothes dryer or apply heat.

18. Is the M-Power™ System a medical device and can it be used to cure disease?

This is an important question. Let's be clear. At Layers of Light International, Inc. we do not diagnose, treat or cure disease. Our M-Power™ products create an environment in your body so that your body can take care of itself through its own innate intelligence.

19. There are many energy products on the market. What separates the M-Power™ Products from the others?

The M-Power™ Products harmonize and organize your bio-energy field to promote higher consciousness. Many of the other energy products manipulate your energy field and may provide short term positive results. For detailed information please refer to the Layers of Light International Position statement regarding The Bio-Energy Crises on our website. **www.2lolii.com/dandyone**

The difference the M-Power Trio has made for me has been so great. I collapsed at work a little over 4 years ago. I was one of the 80 to 90 percent of people who wind up in the hospital for a stress related illness. The stress caught up to me and I began having panic attacks, acute anxiety and TIA's. After collapsing, I could not walk without holding on to the walls. It was necessary for me to crawl up the stairs. There was some improvement in my balance and learned a new way of thinking.

Within the first day I noticed a big shift. In the last 10 months of using the system, I have had no panic attacks, anxiety or TIA's.

I went to my first yoga class. The teacher said I was a natural. **My balance has improved.**

I thought I was really positive before. Affirmations were my way of life. I didn't realize that negative thoughts were not only buried, but when a negative thought appeared, I cancelled it instantly and replaced it with a positive. I noticed that **my negative thoughts were not surfacing** and noticed an actual void in my thoughts. It was a weird feeling until **I started replacing the void with exciting thoughts and desires**. This will surely accelerate my success.

LAYERS of LIGHT INTERNATIONAL, INC.
www.2lolii.com/dandyone

What you can experience:
1. Improve your Physical Performance: *Balance, Coordination, Flexibility, Strength, & Endurance*
2. Improve your Mental Performance by 30-50% in minutes.
3. Change the Acids to Alkalinity in minutes.
4. Optimize the Oxygenization of the body Systems in minutes.
5. Increase Brain Stimulation & Balancing.
6. Increase Cellular Life Extension.
7. Enhance your Performance Outcomes.
8. Increase your energy.
9. Erase your Excessive Stress.
10. Block the damaging Frequencies of Cell & Mobile Phones

"Clinical and in numerous laboratory experiments and studies have Dr. Hans Selye of the University of Montreal has proved the existence of a basic life force, which he call "adaptation energy.'
86

Throughout life we are daily called on to adapt to stressful situations. Even the process of living itself constitutes stress—or continual adaptation. Dr. Selye found the human body contains various defense mechanisms (local adaptation syndromes or LAS), which defend against specific stress, and a general defense mechanism (general adaptation syndrome or GAS), which defend against nonspecific stress. "Stress" includes anything that requires adaptation or adjustment such as extremes of heat or cold, invasion by disease germs, emotional tension, the wear and tear of living, or the so-called aging process. (As any of the tension of 600 muscles, tendons, or ligaments are released from the stressors, the spine and body systems go out of alignment and we usually suffer pain and/or inflammation.)

"This "adaptation energy" is something different from the caloric energy we receive from food. . . . The really important things that Dr. Selye has proved is that the body itself is equipped to maintain itself in health, to cure itself of disease, and to remain youthful by successfully coping with those factors that bring about what we call old age (if we correct the stressors). Not only has he proved that the body is capable of curing itself, but that in the final analysis that is the only sort of cure there is. *Various therapies work largely by either stimulating the body's own defense mechanism when it is deficient, or toning it down when it is excessive.* The adaptation energy itself is what finally overcomes the disease, heals the wound or burn, or wins out over other stressors."(According to Quantum Physicists when the body becomes overstressed it goes into a back up energy system in which any and up to 600 muscles are released. As a result, if this system fails, the body also has a tertiary back up system.)

"Is This the Secret of Youth?

"This élan vital, life force, or adaptation energy manifests itself in many ways. This energy that heals a wound is the same energy that keeps all our body organs functioning. When this energy is at an optimum level all our organs function better, we feel good, wounds heal faster, we are more resistant to disease, we recover from any sort of stress faster, we feel and act younger, and in fact biologically we are younger. It is possible to correlate the various manifestations

87

of this life force and to assume that whatever works to make more of this life force available to us, whatever opens to us a greater influx of life stuff, whatever helps us utilize it better—helps us all over."

"We may conclude that whatever nonspecific therapy aids wounds to heal faster might also make us feel younger. Whatever nonspecific therapy helps us overcome aches and pains might, for example, extend physical life and improve quality of life. One can be intrigued with the increase of mental, and psychological factors. And this is precisely the direction that medical research is now taking. This appears most promising.

Dr. Sari Y. Suttka, D.C. is a renowned expert in Sports Medicine who is known to achieve peak performance in elite athletes. She did preliminary work with Dr. Ronald H. Jones (one of the pioneers in the early applications of MRI and many other medical products) and has conducted studies regarding the effects of vibrations, frequencies, and tones on healing. Specifically, she has been studying the use of various forms of inorganic, organic, and musical tones to see which will achieve and maintain a high level of coherent balance of energy flow in the human body. There are clinical studies on patient demographic embracing pediatrics to geriatrics, which include over 200 major medical disorders. She has been studying the healing effects of sound and special frequencies for decades. Certain inorganic and organic crystals with specialized frequencies as well as music can obtain and sustain Optimum Center of Energy and Optimum Center of Gravity.

Jeff Gaal speaks

"Everywhere there is energy. If you have ever taken a magnet and put it close to your computer screen or TV, it gets distorted. That is a subtle energy interrupter. This same thing happens to your physical body. The energy field exists around you physically, around your body. So what Layers of Light has identified is that there are so many of these energy interrupters that they have completely manipulated your energy and this manifests physical conditions, meaning un-wellness or poor quality of life,. So let's look at what these energy interrupters do. First, the 80,000 man made chemicals in the air you breath, the food you eat, and the
88

water you drink. Those you can't hide from. They are part of your everyday life. Those are energy interrupters. A good visual of how it affects our body is a river flowing with water. That represents our energy. There is an even flow of energy. If you take a rock and place that rock in the middle of the river, what happens? It divides the flow of water like the flow of energy causing eddies and whirlpools that swish around. Imagine now, the man made chemicals in the air as rocks in your river of flowing energy. There is a great web site you can go to: www.ewg.org. That is an environmentally working group and is a great 3rd party reference. You will get some education on what we are talking about.

Secondly, gravity presents a tremendous problem. Gravity affects you. It keeps you on the earth, but it has a negative effect on your body. As we age we walk with small strides, we are hunched over, and get saggy: All from the effects of gravity. Then, there is electro-pollution (EMF), all the things that have a current running through them: TV, radio, cell phones, anything in your house electrical, hair dryers. All of these things manipulate your energy fields. Then you have metals, scars, tattoos and piercing. All of these are rocks in your river of energy.

Probably the biggest energy interrupters are our negative thoughts. Imagine the river that was once empty is now full of thousands of rocks. What's happening to your energy flow? What happens to the water? It's completely disrupted. There is no flow. It's all over the place and we believe that it manifests into physical conditions and a state of un-wellness.

So what Layers of Light does, very simply, is to remove the rocks from your river, your energy interrupters which allows your energy to realign more evenly, without you knowing any interruptions from your body. It is self-adjusting where it will actually repair itself. How do we know this? If you break a limb, you go to the doctor. Does the doctor actually repair your arm? Not really. He puts it in a cast and creates an environment so your body begins to heal itself. It is auto poetic, it is self-adjusting. The same thing happens when we remove that energy interrupter; the body begins to heal itself. So how do we do it? We do it with what we call fusion formulas.

Fusion Formulas take the best of Eastern Medicine and the best of Western Medicine and attach it to energy. We provide 3 products in a system and energy is imbued into these products as carriers or holders of that energy. Dr. Sarri Suttka developed these products and has over 12 years experience with elite athletics, understanding energy and how the body works, and how interrupters work on the body. So what we have done is developed a set of products from products that you consume: something you wear, something you spray into your field around you and something you ingest. What this does is remove the energy interrupters.

What that means to you; what is in it for you; what we guarantee is an immediate increase of 5 physical factors: Performance, Strength, Balance, Coordination, and Flexibility. Along with this we begin to see an increase in Mental Clarity and Focus. Along with that is a lot of auto poetic, self adjusting. Though we do not make any medical claims we have a lot of testimonies of the body doing self repair from Lupus, MS, Fibromyalgia, Chronic Fatigue, Seizures, Arthritis, High Blood Pressure, High Cholesterol, The body does it to repair itself. That is what our Company does. That is the product that we deliver. Do you have any questions at this time?

How do you take the product to get results?

Conference Call: Jan 21, 2004
Dr. Suttka, can you tell us a little about your background and what got you to this point?
In 1991 I began experimenting with ultrasound, oils, crystals (which, of course are in the ultrasound machines) and looking at pain inflammation and the connective tissues. All of that research works with crystals. I don't know if you know this, but crystals are in the sound track of an ultrasound. That was my first exposure to manifesting electrical energy to mechanical energy through a crystal.

That led to an application for a patent in 1994. I started mass-producing oil that I had developed and a pharmaceutical company was going to fund research for it. The head or the director of the pharmaceutical company wanted to make sure that my claims were valid, so he took the oils to Dr. Ronald H. Jones. He introduced me
90

to this wonderful world of energy. Mr. Jones was actually a consultant with this company. He would look at medical devices, medical discoveries and basically do some research and then give his opinion whether it was true or not.

So an ultrasound is a crystal in a tube or wand or something, and you put electricity through the crystal?

Yes, I found that doctors have different machines with different crystals in them and were getting different results and it was based upon the crystal inside or surface area So I saw a direct connection between the surface area and the amount of energy produced. That is why I came up with the energy pouch the way it is. The crystals have a surface area and that's why they are crushed to a certain size.

"We did a test on a 30 year old patient with congenital heart problems since birth. She had had open-heart surgery when she was 3 years old, 7 years old and was still having problems. Using an Acoustic Cardiograph, you could see on the chart that the heart was very, very weak The amplitude between the beats was very low, there was very little resting in between one beat and another beat. When we took the Pouch away and added the music, the amplitude jumped a very little bit, but the resting in between was remarkable. It just calmed her down. The music calmed her down almost instantaneously. When we added the Energy Pouch and music together it was almost like a perfectly normal heart. The amplitude was very strong which shows that the heart was stronger. The resting amplitude increased twice as much as it did from the baseline. She had more noise in between each beat (which told me that she wasn't resting, which gave her more energy to the heart). That instantaneous change that happened to the heart really impressed me greatly.

Have you done a lot with sports medicine?

"Yes, I was the performance consultant for the American cup Team in 1995. Back in 1991 when I first started working with this experimental program I began working with the effects of gravity. Optimal Center of Gravity was what I had achieved to a point that what I called Power Peds, developed in the early 90's. Those Power

Peds went into the American Cup Team, the first female competitors and they almost owned the race. We saw tremendous increases in endurance and strength. That was the beginning of what we see today.

Explain what you mean by Optimal Center of Gravity?

We have a force that is always working upon us: downward – gravity. So we have a Center of Mass at the body about 2 inches below the navel – your Center of Mass. When the optimal Center of Gravity and the Center of Mass are out of alignment you need to expend more energy just to stand upright. That is not even considering movement, so when you begin to move in coordination 600 muscles set fire to the brain for their position. If this force of gravity and the Center of Mass are not in alignment, you are going to expend more energy just standing, let alone considering moving. When those two forces are in alignment that is when you see increased strength, increased flexibility, endurance and all these factors that we look at."

How do they get out of alignment?

There are so many things, the food we eat, the air we breathe, toxins, electromagnetic frequencies (EMF). All of those interrupt the body's electromagnetic field externally as well as internally. So all of these forces, all of what I call "interference patterns" (stress) that's what they do is set up interference patterns and your body starts to get cold and muscles go weak. The body starts to torque and we lose our flexibility and so forth.

So the power and the frequencies in your products help to realign these patterns?

It creates what I call a "coherent" or a "reference wave" and everything starts into an energy with that wave. That wave took a long time to identify, but what we see immediately when we put the pouch on or listen to the music or take the matrix, there is a coherent pattern developing. We saw on a brain map, that the body is going toward its optimal state of coherent energy. The pouch and the JAS

92

energy give us a map, which the body then models. I like to think of it as a reference wave to harmony or wellness.

I began the work with Optimal Center of Gravity in 1991 and then met Dr. Jones in 1994. We developed the pouch with the crystals, which came out in 1996. Then we met Robert Aviles & introduced the JAS energy through his music, which can reach the environment because we were very limited at the time working with just the crystals... and the Energy Mix is something Dr. Jones had developed. So now we needed to address the environment.

What do you mean by "addressing the environment?

"All of the inharmonious frequencies that we are exposed to during the day in the house. Look around you . . . you have florescent lighting. They say we live in a toxic environment . . .it is more toxic inside than it is outside! All the chemicals we are exposed to, electromagnetic fields, air pollution, gravity, negative thoughts and emotions of people around you, radiation from nuclear plants, aromatherapy in cleaning products, metal fillings, implants toxins, even one's own negative thoughts and emotions, etc. Getting in a shower is toxic . . . there are so many things that surround us. Many people don't know this, but chlorine above 75 degrees becomes chloroform, so take a cold shower these days!

"The music not only addresses the environment, it works to create the harmonious systems in the body as well. The pouch is a different method of bringing frequencies to the body. It has its own crystalline base structure, which creates this harmonic, so when you put it on a person you get to see all of these effects. We have measured that it is a dose-related effect and we have done several studies to show this brain mapping and other reactions. Just the pouch by itself is one-third of the system, so you do not get the harmonics of the full system until you add the other two. A very apparent test was when we put the pouch on a person doing an acoustic cardiogram, and we saw that the electrical conductors of the heart really become strong, so there was a lot of energy going into the heart, but what the music did was calm the heart.

Would these products protect you from the EMF's of the environment?

"The pouch, the mix, and the spray work together to protect you within a certain band of frequencies on a continuum of inharmonics. We are addressing just a small band of the ultimate toxic frequencies that are out there today. We have gamma rays, we have x-rays (by the way x-rays come out of florescent tubes (I don't know whether you know it or not). We have higher frequencies that the system does not protect you against. That's why we have been doing research for several years now on the Soma tones. That is an extension of the Life System and it will be coming out soon.

We hear a variety of different "frequency" products on the market. There is even a company that supposedly is programming computer chips with certain frequencies and strapping them to certain parts of the body. How does that sort of thing compare?

"It is so simplistic to think one thing can do it all when you understand all of the inharmonics and all of the chemicals that are out there. There are over 80,0000 man-made chemicals, and to think you could just do one little thing on the body that is going to make bacteria in your gut! I don't think so. That's why this is a system. The Q-Power Marine Matrix is so important because that goes into the gut to create a flora, an internal environment that creates your B vitamins and B vitamins are necessary to make energy. It writes those energy cycles and it also makes chemicals to break down cholesterol. How is a chip going to do that?

"We need to address the environment in which we live, as well as the internal environment. That's the highest frequency of all. So that is the progression of the Life System, and then going into the Soma tones, because to create wellness, we needed to address all of these frequencies. It is not simplistic. I wish it were. It is very complex.

"We are not just this physical body, we are multi-dimensional beings and we need to have interference to these multi-dimensions when we begin working with the physical body and its counterparts. This system addresses these multi-dimensional levels as well as the physical body.

94

Are you able to test these products that resonate with the body?

"Dr. Debbie Crews, Assistant Research Professor at Arizona State University is world renowned for brain mapping. She has completed segments on 20/20 with Alan Alda just recently on brain mapping for Scientific American Journal. She was doing some brain mapping using the product. She said, "Oh, my gosh! This is something that I haven't seen but a few times in my 20 years of brain mapping." When an athlete is in their peak performance and they are doing everything perfectly I see a wave called Theta wave. Theta wave in the brain is where the entire format starts a synergy to the Theta wave and the Theta wave is very similar to meditation. You wouldn't think a person who is meditating is at their highest physical performance, but it's in that zone where they're calm, they're focused, they're clear, they don't have any stress and their performance is at a peak.

"In the case study, we looked at individuals in a resting state, the baseline, to see the amount of activity in the brain. The mount of activity is represented by the brightness of the colors on the brain map. Second, we looked for the balance of the two hemispheres of the brain, looking at eight different sites. The maps indicate four different frequency bands which represent different types of activity. Theta, Alpha, Beta, and Beta II. The amount of activity is important to look at and it is obvious in the baseline that there was limited imbalance, especially in Beta and Alpha. Beta had very little activity.

So this thing is about vibratory elevation or vibratory correcting moving into a state of harmony.

"The mission of the company is to transform hate to love and we are starting to see it in those Soma tone maps. It's a state of clearness and clarity. In developing products for humans, there are seven energy bridges in the brain and a connecting bridge. Each of these energy bridges has seven sub bridges.

Have you done any studies with animals?

"You know, pets have very similar problems to their owners. But animals only have three energy bridges. They had a few that were neurotic, had allergies, had energy brain-outs, barking anxiety, tumors, etc. Within the two weeks all eight dogs were normalized. Their neurosis went away, one dog had a disk problem and that went away, their allergies were gone, and the owners know their pets and they all said they noticed major differences in their dogs' habits of eating and exercising. All we did was put the pouch on and give them the Q-Power Marine Matrix according to the dog's state at that time. Some dogs were very sick and we recommended a little bit more. A couple of dogs had cancer and so forth. That's all they did, put the energy pouch on their collar and fed them the Marine Matrix. They had a 100% success rate with the animals."

SUGAR

I was planning to write a little on sugar. I think just about everyone knows that sugar is a thing to avoid. Yet almost everyone knows also that glucose (a sugar) is fed intravenously to those who are in the hospital unable to eat. This is actually done to keep the patient alive. So how could sugar be so bad for us. It is and yet it isn't. There are many forms of sugar.

The reason that I am not going in to it is because R. Neil Voss has graciously given me the findings of his research. It is technical and lengthy. I was planning to abridge it but it is so full of great information. It should be of interested to those technical people and those who just want to be informed.

This is the only part of the book that encourages you to avoid something. It is a do book but I encourage avoidance on excess short chain sugar intake. If you can avoid the unhealthy sugars completely, you could very well be better off. The following 35 pages are the findings of his report.

SECTION TWO
R. NEIL VOSS, RESEARCHER
American Fork, UT 84003 www.vossenergy@aol.com

WHY CERTAIN FOODS WILL CAUSE 60% of the POPULATION to get DIABETES and 33% to get CANCER!

THE SECRET TO THE NEW EPIDEMIC - DIABETES

Researchers have found that 60% of the population in America will get Diabetes some time in their life. It appears that 18 million American have diabetes, and that 5.2 million are unaware they have the disease according to the Diabetic Association. Beyond this there are another 20.1 million Americans who have a pre-diabetic condition that involves higher than normal glucose levels, but haven't yet had a type-2 diabetic diagnosis.

How did we end up with what medical professionals are calling a full-blown epidemic?

DIABETES BEGINS WITH HYPOGLYCEMIA

Researchers have found that diabetes starts with hypoglycemia (Low blood sugar). It is sometimes eight years or more of Hypoglycemia before one is diagnosed. Researchers find about 100 Million people have hypoglycemia (Dr. David Williams – Hypoglycemia: The Deadly Roller Coaster. "The low blood sugar of today is the diabetes of tomorrow" (Seale Harris, M.D.) What is it and how can we protect ourselves?

"In simple layman's language, hypoglycemia is the body's inability to properly handle the large amounts of glucose and fructose sugars that the average American consumes today. It's an overload of sugar, sugar cereals, refined carbohydrates, alcohol, caffeine, soda drinks, sweetened drinks and (the wrong) foods combined with stress."

"In medical terms, hypoglycemia is defined in relation to its causes. Hypoglycemia is the over secretion of insulin by the pancreas in response to a rapid rise in blood sugar, too many glucose sugars, fructose, or the cells in the body becoming insulin resistant.

"Your blood sugar can drop for many reasons, including skipping a meal, exercising more strenuously than normal, not adjusting your medication." The body needs energy in the form a glycogen from the liver about every 4-5 hours. Under normal circumstances watch eating between meals as you will disturb the manufacturing process taking place in the liver to create energy for the cells.'

Many people are wondering why certain nutrition, vitamins, minerals, and certain nutrients are not working in their body? "A summary of some of the symptoms of hypoglycemia are:

fatigue	faintness	heart palpitations	mood swings
sweating	nausea	hunger	mental confusion
Insomnia	headaches	craving for sweets	dizziness
Depression	allergies	cold hands & feet	blurred vision
nervousness	forgetfulness	crying spells	trembling
Confusion	weakness	drowsiness	outburst of temper

Once you reach the stage of diabetes here are some things that are happening.

* "High blood sugar (diabetic hyperosmolar syndrome) causes your blood sugar to become so high that your blood actually becomes thick and syrupy, mainly in type 2 diabetes."

* "Increased blood acids (diabetic ketoacidosis) sometimes cause your cells to become so starved for energy that the body begins to break down, producing toxic acids known a ketones, mostly type 1 diabetes. The signs and symptoms – include loss of appetite, nausea, vomiting, fever, stomach pain and a sweet, fruity smell on your breath – sometimes mistaken for the flu."

Long-term complications

* "Nerve damage (neuropathy) happens to about 50% of all people with diabetes. This occurs because excess sugar injures the walls of the tiny blood vessels (capillaries) that nourish the nerves. The
98

symptoms depend on which nerves are affected." When the nerves die, the muscles begin wasting away, because there is no mechanism to send messages that the muscles need food. (Dr. Stephen Berry)

* "Sugar damages the sensory nerves in the legs and arms. This causes tingling, numbness, burning or pain that usually begins at the tips of the toes or fingers and over a period of months or years gradually spreads upwards. Because you may not feel any discomfort in your feet, you may develop vascular problems such as skin ulcers and open sores. In addition, damage to the nerves that control digestion can cause problems with nausea, vomiting, diarrhea, or constipation."

* "Kidney damage (nephropathy) is created when the millions of tiny blood vessels that filter waste from your blood and eliminate it in the urine become damaged. By the time symptoms appear, ankles, feet and hands are swollen, anemia, shortness of breath, and high blood pressure, and extensive nerve and kidney damage."

* "Eye damage (retinopathy) happens to type 1 and type 2 Diabetes because of the deterioration in the blood vessels of the retina."

* "Diabetes leads to cataracts and a greater risk of glaucoma. Diabetes is the leading cause of blindness in the United States."

HEART PROBLEMS WILL HIT 1 IN 4

* "Heart and blood vessel (cardiovascular disease) dramatically increases your risk, including chest pain (angina), heart attack, stroke, narrowing of the arteries (arteriosclerosis) and high blood pressure. Usually there are also raised blood levels of triglycerides and lower levels of high-density lipoprotein ((HDL) – the "good" cholesterol that may protect against heart disease."

* "Infection happens when high blood sugar impairs the immune system. The mouth, gums, lungs, skin, feet, kidneys, bladder, and genital areas are all susceptible to infection." (Brown, S)

WHY EYE PROBLEMS DEVELOP

"The lens has a crystalline structure made of protein fiber. The perfect operation of the lens requires normal concentrations of sodium, potassium, protein, and calcium. These levels are maintained by the sodium-potassium pump, which is a sulphur containing protein. As you age, more sodium remains in the lens and less potassium gets into it. This imbalance makes the fiber (of protein) clump together (much the same process that turns an egg white from clear to white during cooking). Older fibers are also pushed to the center of the lens. The clumping and pushing causes the lens to cloud over causing cataracts."

SECRETS TO COMBINING THE NECESSARY BUILDING BLOCKS FOR THE BODY

The body does not as an end result create just Proteins (Amino Acids), Sugars (Mono & Polysaccharides), Carbohydrates, and Fatty Acids, but the end result of all of these building blocks create chains of **GLYCOPROTEINS (Sugar molecules + Proteins molecules), GLYCOLIPIDS (Sugar molecules + Fat molecules), and Proteolysis (1 Protein molecule, Sugar molecules) + Carbohydrates). Glyco-proteins are the most abundantly produced building blocks in the body. Next, are the Glyco-lipids. There are limited carbohydrates used in the body.**

FRUITS AND VEGETABLE IN THE AMERICAN DIET: NHANES II SURVEY

Health and Nutrition Examination Survey (1976-80):
1. 45% of the population ate no fruits or vegetables or juice.
2. 27% had no fruit.
3. 22% had no vegetables.
4. 29% had 2 servings of fruit
5. 27% had 2 servings of fruits and vegetables.

It has been recommended to have 5-9 servings of fruits and vegetables.

WHY are GLYCOPROTEINS (Combinations of large numbers of Amino Acids mixed with Sugars) the MOST ABUNDANT BUILDING BLOCKS in the BODY?

"The body has no mechanism for storing protein. If you don't get an adequate amount of energy in the diet then the body protein (be broken down and) will be converted to amino acids that will be used for energy production and the nitrogen will be lost. When too much nitrogen is lost (more is processed than taken in), you will be in a state of negative nitrogen balance, no matter how high the quality of protein. (The body cannot make protein without nitrogen and sulfur. Where do you get nitrogen? dark green vegetables.) When protein from these sources is eaten by itself, without all of the amino acids found in the greens, protein cannot be used to replenish body protein. The mixture after digestion and absorption will be limited with missing amino acids. When the body tries to synthesize proteins, it will run out of amino acids first and essential proteins can't be made." (University of Victoria)

There appears to be over 100,000 different proteins that your body produces. "The DNA determines the order of amino acids in the proteins the organism is capable of making. The order of amino acids for each protein determines its final three-dimensional shape, which in turn determines the function of that protein." The following is a list of approximately 80 to 90 known proteins: **AA protein** (amyloid), **acute phase protein** (found in the serum; they include C-reactive protein), **serum amyloid protein** (A protein, fibrinogen and an acid glycol-proteins), **AL protein** (amyloid light chain), **alcohol-soluble protein** (Prolamin), **Amyloid A proteins** (occurring in reactive systemic fever), **amyloid light chanin proteins** (occurring in immunocyte and immunoglobulin derivation functions), **bactericidal permeability increasing proteins** (a cationic antibacterial protein occurring in neutrophil granules), **Bence Jones protein** (Urinary protein), binding protein (binds and transports other substances, such as ions, sugar, nucleic acids, or amino acids, **bone Gla protein** ((osteocalcin), **bone morphogenetic protein** (stimulates osteogenesis), **protein C** (forms clotting in plasma), **CAD protein** (catalytic for 3 enzymes), **carrier protein** (causes happen to elicit an immune response), **C4 binding protein** (a complement system regulator protein), **coagulated protein** (an insoluble form created when denatured by heat, alcohol, ultraviolet rays, or chemical agents.), **complement control protein** (a super family of proteins regulating gene clusters), **complete protein** (as apposed to partial proteins), **compound proteins or conjugate proteins** (linked to other building blocks, e.g. Salty proteins, nucleoproteins, glycol-proteins, glycol-lipids, metallo-proteins, homo-proteins, chromo-proteins, hemo-proteins, and phos-proteins), **constitutive proteins, cord proteins** (blood from the umbilical cord), **C-reactive proteins** (globulin), **cystic fibrosis trans-membrane regulator proteins, decay accelerating factor proteins, derived protein** (formed by hydrolyte changes – peptones, peptides), **encephalitogenic proteins** (myelin), **fibrillar protein or fibrous proteins** (collagens, elastins, keratins, actins, and myosin), **functional proteins** (hemoglobin, insulin, and other activities and functions), **fusion protein** (produced by the genes of the DNA), **G proteins** (intracellular functions with receptors), **glial fibrillary acidic proteins** (forming the glial filaments of the astrocytes), **GM activator proteins** (sphingolipid activator), **GTP activating protein** (regulates G, GTP binding, GDP proteins), **guaranyl-nucleotide binding protein, H proteins, immune protein** (immunoglobulin), **incomplete proteins** (protein without the complete ratio of amino acids different than necessary), **insoluble protein** (a substance left behind after the other proteins have been extracted from the cell), **iron-sulfur protein** (function for electron transport), **leukocyte adhesion proteins** (integrin), **maintenance proteins, major basic proteins** (a cationic protein in eosinophic granules have cytotoxic activity against my parasites), **membrane protein** (membranes of enzyme, receptor for a hormone or other molecules, lipid-insoluble substances, **Membrane cofactor protein** (transport of substances across the plasma), **myelin basic protein** (encephalomyelitis by inducing T cell activity that leads to demyelinization and lymphoid infiltration), **myeloma protein** (immunoglobulin proteins), **myosin protein** (occurs in the muscle tissue-ability of muscles to contract), **native protein, parathyroid hormone-like protein, parathyroid hormone-related protein, plasma proteins, Pot1 proteins** (cap the chromosomes so telomerase regulation is correct),**prion protein, proteolopid protein** (major constituent of myelin in the central nervous system), **R protein** (rapid electrophoretic mobility relative to intrinsic factor-

102

carbon atom), **racemized protein** (proteins changed by chemical or other agents), **recombinant protein** (involved in ability to produce gene product), **retinal binding protein** (a-globulin synthesized and secreted by the liver), **protein diasulfide isomerase, protein glutamine, protein kinase, protein S** (plasma protein inhibits blood clotting), **RNAs P protein** (a RNA cutting molecule), **S protein** (not protein S), **S-100 protein** (protein in the central nervous system and ganglia, **serum proteins** (blood serum plasma), **serum amyloid A protein** (suppresses antibody responses), **simple proteins** (complete amino acids on complete hydrolysis), **sphingolipid activator protein, staphylococcal protein A, Structural proteins** (keratin, collagen for hair, muscles, tendons, and skin), **telomere proteins** (that cap the chromosome ends of DNA), **transport protein, whole protein, zinc finger proteins."** You can see how important proteins are and how many there are beyond this list. Some when combined with different sugars are 10,000, 20,000, and 30,000 molecules long folded up.

WHAT IF YOU DO NOT GET ENOUGH PROTEIN TO MAKE TELOMERAE PROTEIN?

"Dr. Zakian found a naturally occurring protein that inhibits the activity of another protein, called telomerse, which replicates and lengthens the very ends of chromosomes. The protein, called Pif1p acts directly on the chromosome ends, called telomerse, to keep the lengthening process in check. Telomerse is present in 90% of cancer types, but is absent from most healthy cells." There are nucleic acid/protein structures that act as caps (on the end of the chromosomes) to prevent the DNA in these chromosomal regions from degrading and from being inappropriately joined together." (Lyons)

WHAT CAUSES THINGS IN THE BODY TO GO AWRY?

"In 1937, the Nobel Prize for medicine was awarded to the father of nutritional science, Dr. Albert Szent Gyorgi, for discovering Vitamin C. He was the first scientist to isolate the active ingredient in oranges and limes. After conducting additional research, the doctor was astonished. He found Vitamin C opened up the capillaries of the blood vessels. He discovered that scurvy patients did not recover as quickly when they were given the simple isolated form of vitamin C as when a whole food complex was given. This disappointed Dr. Szent Gyorgi because he was confident he had found an efficient way to cure this disease."

In his speech to the Nobel Prize Committee Szent Gyorgi warned that the single isolated chemical Vitamin was not as effective as whole food."

"Dr. Szent Gyorgi focused his scientific research on discovering the other compound in whole food that make it effective. Before his death in 1986 he discovered a variety of biologically active substances including flavin and flavonone (Vitamin P)."

"In 1999, Dr. Gunter Blobel was awarded a Nobel Prize for his research when he discovered the exact mechanisms of how nutrients are transported into the cells of our bodies. He discovered this amazing information after spending 20 years researching just one question, "How do proteins know where to go in the body?"

"It was discovered that nutrients inside food are bound by many other essential elements, such as amino acids, sugars, and lipids (fats), which are called carrier co-factors. The most important of these cofactors are the proteins. These proteins were discovered to contain unique signals that act like a zip code to transport the attached nutrients to the cells that need them."

"These proteins are called protein chaperones because they take nutrients to the cells with them. There are many different protein chaperones, depending on which vitamin or mineral needs to be transported to which of the various cells." These proteins work in conjunction with Glutithione, which is a transporter and recycler of amino acids and nutrients."

If you want calcium to get into your bones, then the calcium you take must have the appropriate protein chaperone attached, otherwise it won't know where to go! The appropriate carrier cofactors must be present for the body to absorb, utilize, and retain all the nutrients bound inside the food."

104

"This was the answer to Dr. Szent Gyorgi's mystery of why ascorbic acid (Vitamin C) did not cure scurvy, but oranges and limes did! Without the attached protein chaperone, and all the other cofactors, the body could not utilize the isolated chemical nutrient (ascorbic acid) well enough to cure scurvy." (Brown)

From the basis of Dr. Gunter Blobel's research, we see why it is important to find nutritional products that are food based to enable the body and it's billions of cells to properly communicate with each other through the balanced use of amino acids, sugars and fat for the proper nutrients to get to the areas of the body that were intended to receive them.

PROTEINS BECOME DENATURED BECAUSE OF TEMPERATURE

"Denaturing can be defined as any modification of the secondary, tertiary, or quaternary structures of the protein molecule, the breakage of covalent bonds. Denaturation is a process by which hydrogen bonds, hydrophobic interactions and salt linkages are broken and the protein (molecules) are unfolded." (Fennema, OR) These molecules are sometimes 200 to 30,000 molecules long.

"The mechanism of temperature-induced denaturation is highly complex and involves primarily destabilization of the major non-covalent interactions. Hydrogen bonding, electrostatic and Van der Waals interactions are exothermic in nature."

"When a protein solution is heated above a critical temperature, it undergoes a sharp transition from the native state to the denatured state. The temperature at the transition midpoint where the concentration ratio of the native product, and the denatured state is either the melting temperature or the denaturation temperature."

"At 40 degrees Centigrade for a period of 10 minutes all of the protein is stable and intact. At 45 degrees Centigrade there is about 15% denaturing of the protein. At 50 degrees there is about 50% denaturing of the protein, and at 66% there is a denaturing of 100% of the protein molecules. At this level the protein molecules (200 to 30,000 long) unwind or unfold." (Scopes, RK)

A good example of this is raw milk. When the raw milk is heated over a temperature of 72 degrees Centigrade, it breaks the bonds that hold the molecules together and the Cystein and Cystine amino acids are destroyed. This is the major reason people are allergic to milk." "A good example of a denatured protein is an egg white that has been cooked above 212 degrees F. The amino acids are still present in a denatured protein," but the proteins become deformed."

MECHANISM OF TEMPERATURE DISTRUCTION

"The mechanism of temperature-induced denaturation is highly complex and involves primarily destabilization of the major non-covalent interactions. Hydrogen bonding, electrostatic, and Van der Waals interactions are exothermic in nature. Therefore, they are destabilized at high temperatures and stabilized at low temperatures."

The research showing the percentage of protein remaining that is not un-denatured after 10 min. incubation starts at 100% at 40 degrees C. At 45 degrees there is about 80% real protein left. At 50 degrees 50% of the real protein is lost. At 55 degrees C. there is virtually no protein left that is un-denatured in the product.

FACTORS AFFECTING THE PROCESSING OF PROTEINS

"Susceptibility of proteins to heat denaturation depends on a number of factors. Water greatly facilitates thermal denaturation of proteins. Dry protein powders are extremely stable to thermal denaturation. (If they have not been overheated previously) The value of the denaturing temperature decreases rapidly as the water content is increased from 0-to 0.35-water/g. protein. An increase in water content from 0.35 to 0.75 g water/g. protein, the temperature denaturation is only a marginal decrease. Above 0.75 water/ g. protein, the temperature denaturation of the protein is the same as in dilute protein solution. Some proteins are stable at temperatures as high as 100 degrees C. if the moisture content is very low." (Scopes)

"Additives such as salts and sugars affect thermo stability of proteins in aqueous solutions. Sugars such as sucrose, lactose, glucose, and glycerol stabilize proteins against thermal denaturation.
106

Addition of 0.5 M NaCl to proteins such as b-lacto globulin, serum albumin, and oat globulin significantly increase their temperature denaturation. The amino acid composition also affects thermal stability of proteins: proteins that contain a greater proportion of hydrophobic amino acid residues, especially."

"Proteins can become denatured with extremes of pH of food and as they unfold and lose the structural organization, the denatured proteins lose their function and their properties can also change, they sometimes become insoluble or change their color."

"Unfortunately, routine metabolic process can damage proteins. For example, when exposed to free radicals, proteins become oxidized, that is, corroded from the inside out. The proteins then rapidly degenerate. If the oxidation is severe, the proteins will become cross-linked, permanently damaging them." (Sitte)

"The combination of oxidation and Glycation produces cells that are characteristic of cellular aging. These carbonyl groups then induce the proteins to break up, destroying their membrane integrity and speeding up cellular death." (Hipkiss)

"The sugars, (carbohydrates, or glycans as they are called) hexose, pentose, mannose, fucose, n-acetylglucosamin, n-acetylgalactosamine, xylose, and n-acteylneuraminic acid are water-soluble. Because they are water soluble these nutrients would be at least partially depleted when cooked in water."

DESTRUCTION OF MEAT PROTEINS CREATE DEFORMED PROTEINS CALLED – "ADVANCED GLYCATION ENDPRODUCTS"

"During the early stages of cooking (30-50 degrees C.), there is an unfolding of peptide chains, formation of relatively unstable cross linkages, and partial denaturation of the sarcoplasmic proteins. These changes cause a tightening of the myofibrillar structure, resulting in toughness and decreased water-holding capacity. (However, the situation will be better if you cook your meats with water and keep the heat below 212 degrees F.) In the latter stages (carmalization), new stable cross linkages are formed in conjunction with denaturation and coagulation of both collagen shrinks at (61-61 degree C. in meat and 45 degrees C. in fish) and softens as the ordered helical structure collapses. The overall result is tenderization of connective tissue and toughening of myofibrillar proteins." (Scopes)

Researchers have found many of the problems with the Lymph are caused from undigested protein, incomplete proteins, or what really is un-denatured protein. We also find that if a person that is lactate intolerant they may only be reacting to the denaturing of the milk or milk whey. From this evidence, we can understand this may be a contributing cause of lymphoma cancer.

WHAT IS THE DIFFERENCE BETWEEN PROTEIN and CARBOHYDRATES?

Carbohydrate molecules are so named because they have a structure of less than 200 molecules. Proteins, on the other hand, have more than 200 molecules to as high as 30,000 known, according to Harper's Biochemistry. Some researchers indicate they may be as long as 100,000 molecules long. In order for protein to be formed from eating, there must be 10 essential amino acids eaten in your diet in order for your body to make protein. If you are sick or stressed, there are an additional 6 amino acids needed in your diet. Your body can create the other 6. The other dietary necessities for making protein are sulfur and nitrogen. You get these by including dark green vegetables in your diet. (Harper's Biochemistry)

GLYCATION OF OUR FOODS

"Eating high temperature cooked foods (above 212 degrees Fahrenheit) is another contributor in the production of inflammation cytokines. In fact, it has been shown that eating these cooked foods leads to the formation of (AGE products). Glycation can be described as the binding of a protein molecule to a glucose molecule resulting in the formation of damaged protein structures. Many age-related diseases such as cataracts, arterial stiffening, neurological impairments, (diabetes, heart problems, skin wrinkles and collagen problems) are attributable to Glycation. These destructive Glycation reactions render proteins in the body cross-linked and barely

108

functional. As these destructive proteins accumulate, they cause cells to emit signals that induce the production of inflammation cytokines." (Life Extension)

"The Inflammatory Cytokine Panel Test should be given to any person suffering from any type of chronic disease to identify the specific inflammatory mediator that is causing or contributing to the disease. Frailty in elderly is linked to Inflammation." (Walston et al. 2002 – Life Extension)

G Proteins, Receptors and Disease

Dr. M. Bumbuli in his Human Biology 101 course teaches, "Adult or late onset (Type II), beta cells function fine, but receptors in target organs begin to malfunction, and are harder to treat. They can only be treated with dietary management and other drugs that help symptoms." http://homepages.bx.edu/~mbumbuli/bio/rev3ans/

"Dr. Fuller Albright began the search concerning many diseases due to an "end-organ to respond to a hormone as from a decrease production or absence of said hormone, in which hormone resistance is a cause of the disease. . . .Fundamental studies on the mechanisms of hormone action culminated in the discovery of a major signal transudation pathway involving heterothimeteric G protein. Hundreds of G-protein-coupled receptors (GPCR), over a dozen G proteins, and a comparable number of effectors regulated by G proteins have now been identified and characterized at the molecular and cellular level. Identification and molecular characterization of these signaling proteins and the genes that encode them allowed them to be tested as candidates responsible for disease of hormone resistance or endocrine hyper function. Many diseases of hormone resistance and of endocrine hyper function are caused by loss-and gain–of-function mutations in G proteins or GPCR. Studies of such diseases, and mutations that cause them, offer unique insights into the relevance, structure and functions of the involved G proteins (All of these G Proteins involve receptors in the cells.)" (Spiegel)

THE MAJOR PROBLEM IN THE BODY IS PROTEIN-SUGAR METABOLISM, PROTEIN-LIPID METABOLISM, AND PROTEIN-CARBOHYDRATE METABOLISM

"The purpose of sugar in the cell is to create (1) sources of carbon and energy and are the (2) structural components of cells (inside and out (3) forming the nucleic acids and (4) the structure of the cell wall." (Van Waasbergen) The body does not just create amino acids from the protein, but mixes the proteins (amino acids in a specific order interspersed with many of 200 sugars. Glycoproteins as they are called are the most abundant proteins made in the body. Next come the Glycolipids."

What are the Foods that Cause the Greatest altering of Proteins and Sugars?

FOOD AGE content u/100 g.
Cooked Animal Skins

(Chicken, Duck, etc.	**6,269,000**	**Free Radical Cells Damaged**
Cake	**836,000**	**Free Radical Cells Damaged**
Pastry	**426,000**	**Free Radical Cells Damaged**
Cereal	**193,400**	**Free Radical Cells Damaged**

BEVERAGES & CONDIMENTS AGE content u/250 ml.

Soy Sauce	**145,027**	**Free Radical Cells Damaged**
Brown Rice Vinegar	**35,007**	**Free Radical Cells Damaged**
Maple Syrup	**13,250**	**Free Radical Cells Damaged**
Diet Coke	**9,600**	**Free Radical Cells Damaged**
Classic Coco-Cola	**8,500**	**Free Radical Cells Damaged**

(Source – Wautier, J.L.)

A LIST of other "AGE"- Advanced glycation end products (deformed sugars & proteins):
Bagels
Bakery Products
Breads
Cereals
Cocoa
110

Coffee Beans, Baked or Roasted
Cooked or Roasted Foods over 212 degrees Fahrenheit
Cookies
Corn Syrups
Crackers
Crusts in Pies
Diet Soda & Cola Drinks
Evaporated Milk
French Fries (100 times the safety limit of Alrylamide)
High Fructose corn syrup
Ice Cream (Filled with foreign food chemicals)
Molasses
Nuts, Roasted Only
Pretzels
Potato Chips – Fried (500 times the safety limit of Alrylamide)
Rolls
Sterilized & Pasteurized Milk Products & Whey (Denatured)
Tortilla Chips
Denatured non-fat yogurts

(Source – Mirkin, Gugliucci)

It has been found that it doesn't matter is it's fried or roasted. If it's heated over 212 degrees Fahrenheit the food creates what is known as Maillardian Reaction. The temperature can be increased if the food is roasted in water and if salt is added to the food.

PROBLEMS WITH MANY DISEASES CAUSED BY PROBLEMS WITH SUGARS

"Many proteins pertinent to normal cell physiology are glycosylated (have sugars attached), and variations in the glycosylation pattern often lead to changes in their function. Most major diseases are associated with a change in the glycosylation pattern of a central protein structure. Axford explored these changes both in health and disease and what the implications are to further understanding disease mechanisms and treatment."

"The altered structures of O Glycans (sugars) may be partly responsible for the pathological properties of diseased cell including cancer, cystic fibrosis, leukemia, inflammatory disease, immune diseases, wound healing, rheumatoid arthritis, Gaucher's disease, hepatitis B, diabetes, heart disease, neurodegenerative diseases, infectious diseases, and other clinical conditions involving cell growth and cell death. It is now understood that there is a 'sugar code' in biological structures that relates to both health and disease."

"The functions of innate immunity are mediated by secreted glycol-proteins and sugar-lectins interactions. Leukocytes, endothelial cells, fibroblasts, phagocytosis, acute phase reactants, protease, cytokines and chemokins are affected by glycol-proteins and sugar-lectin interactions. The basic structure of an IgG antibody molecule is activated by glycol forms (sugars & protein). Autoimmune diseases show a lack of Galactose, mannose, and N-acetylglucosamine." (Axford)

WHAT ARE THE OTHER MAILLARDIAN REACTIONS TO FOODS THAT CAUSE ADVANCED GLYCATION END PRODUCTS IN PROTEINS?

"The Maillard reaction, a browning reaction, happens with any sugar. Fructose browns food more readily (Maillard reaction) than with glucose. This may seem like a good idea, but it is not. With fructose it happens seven times faster than glucose, resulting in a decrease in protein quality and a toxicity of protein in the body. This is due to the loss of amino acid residues and decreased protein digestibility. Many doctors recommend fructose instead of glucose for diabetics. Fructose has no enzymes, vitamins, and minerals and robs the body of its micronutrient treasures in order to assimilate itself for physiological use." (Bunn)

"Research shows that fructose causes a general increase in total serum cholesterol and in the low density lipoproteins (LDL) putting a person at risk of heart disease. There is a significant increase in the concentration of uric acid. An increase in uric acid is an indicator of gout causing preexisting acidotic conditions such as diabetes, postoperative stress, or uremia." (Hallfrisch)

"Fructose is absorbed primarily in the jejunum and metabolized in the liver. It is converted to fatty acids by the liver at a greater rate than is glucose and when the liver cannot convert all of the excess fructose it may be mal-absorbed. What escapes conversion may be thrown out in the urine. Diarrhea can be a consequence. The presence of diarrhea might be the cause of decreased absorption of minerals. Fructose interacts with oral contraceptives and elevates insulin levels in women on the pill. Fructose reduced the affinity of insulin for its receptor." (Zakim)

"Fructose consistently produced higher kidney calcium concentration than did glucose in studies. Fructose generally induced greater urinary concentration of phosphorus and magnesium and lowered urinary pH compared with glucose. Fructose-fed subjects had higher fecal exceptions of iron; calcium, zinc and magnesium than did subjects fed sucrose. A study of 25 patients with functional bowel disease showed that pronounced gastrointestinal distress may be provoked by mal-absorbtion of fructose." (Rumessen)

"Scientists found that the rats given fructose had more undesirable cross linking changes in the collagen of their skin and it may have altered intracellular metabolism. Fructose converts to fat more than any other sugar. Fructose raises serum triglycerides significantly. As a left-handed sugar, fructose digestion is very low. For complete internal conversion into glucose and acetates, it must rob ATP energy stores from the liver. Fructose inhibits copper metabolism. A deficiency in copper leads to bone fragility, anemia, defects of the connective tissue, arteries, and bone, infertility, heart arrhythmias, high cholesterol levels, heart attacks, and an inability to control blood sugar levels."

"It seems that the magnitude of deleterious effects varies depending on such factors as age, sex, baseline glucose, insulin, and triglyceride concentrations, the presence of insulin resistance, and the amount of dietary fructose consumed. Some people are more sensitive to fructose. They include hypertensive, hyperinsulinemic, hypertrigyceridemic, non-insulin dependent diabetic people, people with functional bowel disease and postmenopausal women."

A PAST EPIDEMIC ZOOMS LARGER - CANCER?

One in three will get Cancer.
WHAT ARE THE CANCEROUS PRODUCING ACRYLAMIDES DOING IN OUR DIET?

"Acryl amide is a polymer that is widely used in the treatment of drinking water. It is manufactured of plastics. It was first evaluated as probably carcinogenic to humans by the International Agency for Research on Cancer. Last April Swedish scientists discovered high levels of acryl amide in a wide range of starch-containing foods that are fried or baked, particularly potato chips, French fries, and crackers. They showed that acryl amide is produced when asparagines (an amino acid) abundant in cereals and grains, is heated above 212 degrees Fahrenheit with either of two sugars, glucose or 2-deoxyglucose. Bruce Ganem is a professor in Cornell University's Department of Chemistry and Biology." (Ganem) (Also-Bradley)

"Research in four countries suggests that French fries and potato chips may be a leading cause of cancer in the Western world. Scientists at the meeting of the World Health organization and the United Nations Food and Agricultural Organization are very concerned about the very high levels of acryl amide in the food supply. (Mirkin) Acryl amides are created when the sugars and proteins are cooked at high temperatures over 100 degrees Centigrade (212 degrees Fahrenheit), particularly fried food. "These high temperatures cause the sugar in potatoes to stick to protein to form acryl amides." "Acryl amides are a class of AGE (Advanced Glycation Endproducts."(Mirkin)

"Asparagine is found at particularly high levels in potatoes and in cereals chips, crisps, and crackers (especially those containing rye flour have been found to have some of the highest acryl amide content."

WHAT KIND OF SUGARS (GOOD) ARE THERE IN THE BODY?
Listing of 22 Polysaccharides Needed in the Diet

There are over 200 different kinds of sugars processed in the body. The first 1 through 10 are essential to cell-to-cell communication and cellular function. Next, there needs to be a balance of long chain sugars (Polysaccharides) and short chain sugars in the diet.

Simple Sugars (1-2 polymer units) (Monosaccharides)
1. **N-Glucose (Natural)**
2. **N-Fructose (Natural)**
3. **Galactose (Natural)**

(L-Glucose, L-Fructose, Sucrose, Denatured Lactose are not Natural Sugars*see below)

"Glucose is the precursor of all Amino Sugars that are the important components of glycol-proteins. The major amino sugars are glucosamine (made from glucose), galactosamine (made from Galactose), and mannosamine (made from mannose). Galactose is needed for the synthesis of lactose, glycol-lipids, proteoglycans, and glycol-proteins. Lack of Pentose leads to impairment of red cell hemolysis." Harper's Biochemistry p.212.

DISACCHARIDES
Disaccharides have two sugar molecules:

Maltose is two molecules of L glucose (synthetic mixed with starch. (Found in Beer)
Sucrose is common table sugar and has one molecule of L glucose (processed) and one molecule of L fructose (processed).

4. **"N Lactose** is milk sugar composed of glucose and Galactose. Its full name is glucopyranose."

Oligosaccharides are a few monosaccharides linked together (3-9 polymer units)
(Maltodextrin, Raffinose, Stachyose, fructoligosaccharides (FOS)
"FOS is composed of L fructose and L Sucrose which are not metabolized by the body like natural simple sugars are. FOS are half as sweet as sucrose, yet not absorbed and have minimal caloric

value. N fructoligosaccharides, on the other hand, occur naturally in bananas, garlic, Jerusalem artichokes and technically are a soluble fiber. FOS is usually mixed with high glucose corn syrup. These are synthetic sugars and starches, maltodextrin, raffinose, stachyose, and FOS) have been designed for various purposes of reducing sweetness for diabetics.

Polysaccharides (Greater than 9 polymer units)

5. **Xylose**
6. **Ribitol**
7. **Fucose**
8. **N-acteylneuraminic (or sialic acid)**
   (Links with Serine or Threonine & Asparagine)
9. **N-acetylglucosamine**
10. **N-acetylglactosamine**
11. **Pentose (DNA function) 12. Ribose (RNA cell division functions)**
13. **Amylopectine**
14. **Rhamnose**
15. **Amylose (5 glucose polymers)16. Arabinose (triggers an increase in NK cells)**
17. **Hemicellulose**
18. **Deoxyribose**
19. **Amylopectin (7 glucose polymers)**
20. **Mannose**

"Polysaccharides contain the following growth factors, hormones, and peptides:
Bombesine (a neuropeptides)3 GRP (Gastrin-releasing peptide)4 substance P (a neuropeptides)5 CGRP (Calcitonin-gene peptide) Cortisol (also a neurotransmitter)
IGF-1 (Insulin-like growth factor-1)IGF-2
EGF (Epidermal growth factor)NGF (nerve growth factor)
PRP (Prolactin-releasing peptide)LHRH (or GnRH, stimulates Progesterone Secretion of LH and FSH)
Peptide YY Peptide histidine methionine
Neuropeptide Y (stimulating appetite)Neurotensine
TSH (stimulating T-3 & T-4 secretionBeta-endorphine (opioid peptide)

TRH (stimulating prolactin=GH=T3)T3 (increase # of estrogen receptors)
GHRF (Growth hormone releasing)ACTH (regulating Cortisol secretion)
Small opioid peptides Benzodiazepine=agonist peptides (neurotransmitters)

(Source: Individual sites on the internet)
"Sugar chains of plasma membrane glycol-proteins and glycol-lipids usually face the outside of the cell. They have roles in cell-to-cell interaction (communication) and signaling, and in forming a protective layer on the surface of some cells." (Scientists have identified over 50 different languages as these cells talk to each other, communicate with the brain, and communicate with each body system and function.)

The most monosaccharides and polysaccharides found in the diet if you were to eat 8-10 vegetables and some fruit recommended by the Cancer Society and the AMA is about 8 – 10 Monosaccharides and polysaccharides. In the Goji berry we are able to find 22 monosaccharides and polysaccharides. There are 4 polysaccharides that are not found in any other known plant on earth. These are the master molecules according to Dr. Earl Mindell that function with the Human Growth Hormones (83).

Dietary Sources of (8) Essential Sugars Needed in our Diet
There are **eight complex carbohydrates (Sugars)** that are **essential sugars** needed in the diet every day. They are called glyco-proteins because they mix with protein and sugars. Their function is to create collagens, mucins (Lubricant agents), transport molecules (transferrin), immunologic molecules, thyroid hormones, Enzyme (alkaline phosphatase), plasma proteins of cold water fish (antifreeze), and lectins (agglutinate cells according to blood type). They are nucleotide sugars." (Harper's Biochemistry) These 8 glyco-proteins are transferred to a new baby at birth, but our present diet only gets only a few of these sugars one is eating a recommend 8-10 fruits per day throughout a lifetime. They are: *
1) *Glucose* – Found in certain vegetables, fruits, starch, cane & beet & sugars, sorghum, raw cereals, legumes, un-denatured milk, mushrooms, yeast, bran, animal liver, dates, raisins, honey,

117

grapes, figs, pineapple, carrots, corn, rice, wheat, potatoes, seeds, plant saps, germinating grains, & muscles.

2) *Galactose* – Found in un-denatured milk products, fruits, and vegetables, leeks, onions, and red cabbage, brussel sprouts, green beans, carrots, un-denatured milk, cauliflower, broccoli, red cabbage, kale, parsley, rhubarb, brussels sprouts, asparagus, and plums.

3) *Mannose* – Found in un-denatured sugar. (Aloe Vera, Rappadura Sugar, plant gums, cantaloupe, carrots, beets, cauliflower, broccoli, kale, parsley, rhubarb, brussel sprouts, red cabbage, asparagus.

4) *Fucose* – Found in fruits, raw honey, Jerusalem artichoke, cane sugar, sweet potatoes, dandelions, roots of dahlias, flaxseed, algae, kelp, wakame.

5) *Xylose* (Pentose)– husks of grain, seeds, spelt, rye, oats (unrolled), carrots, beets, cauliflower, broccoli, kale, parsley, rhubarb, brussel sprouts, red cabbage, asparagus, rice, spelt, undenatured milk, germinated grains, & malt.

6) **N-Acteylneuraminic Acid (Sialic acid)** –un-denatured milk, natural hens eggs, un-denatured whey.

7) N-Acetylgalactosamine – un-denatured milk.

8) **N-Acetylglucosamine** – Found in crustaceans, seeds, undenatured milk, algae, tempeh, plant saps, shitake mushroom

9) Glucosamine – Found in yeasts, some algae, fungi, & tempeh.

10) Arabinose – Found in spelt, rye, oats, barley, leeks, carrots, tomatoes, radishes, pears, larch, acacia, corn, seed gums, un-denatured milk, legumes

11) Rhamnose – Seeds & plant saps.

12) *Fructose* (Not High Fructose Corn Syrup)– Most fruits and vegetables, cane, beet sugar, sorghum, seeds, wheat, bran, onion, leeks, artichokes, asparagus, bananas, garlic, grasses, carrots, rice, spelt, germinated grains, mushrooms, cauliflower, broccoli, kale, red lettuce, parsley, rhubarb, brussel sprouts, pineapple, plant gums. "GlycoScience.com"

A. Cue SW, "Polysaccharide Gums from Agricultural Products Edition", Lancaster, Pa: Technomic Publishing Co, Inc, 2001

B.   Budavari S, O'Neil MJ, Smith, A, et al. ed. "the Merch Index, 12th Edition, Whitehouse Station, NJ: Merck & Co., Inc. 1996

C. Chaubey M, KapoorVP. "Structure of a galactomannan from the seeds of Cassia Angustifolia Vahl. Carbohydrates Res 2001, 332 (4): 439-444.

D. Kapoor VP, Taravel FR, Joseleau JP, et al. "Cassia Spectabulin DC seed galacomannan, structural, crystallographical and rheological studies, Carbohydrates Res. 1998;306(1-2) 231-241

E. Liener IE

* Most important in the body. " Too much Glucose correlates with Cancer."

"Conscious Eating," Gabriel Cousens, M.D., pp.77-79. "Harper's Biochemistry" Chapter 56 – Glycoproteins. The sugar Fructose is not a natural sugar and is not the same as the natural sugar Fucose. One can get 6 of these 8 Glycoproteins in un-denatured Whey (Immunocal) also.

An example of the sugars in foods as follows:

Broccoli has uronic acid, arabinose, galactose, xylose, mannose, and fucose.

Cauliflower has uronic acid, arabinose, galactose, xylose, mannose, and fucose.

Carrots have uronic acid, galactose, arabinose, mannose, xylose, and rhamnose.

WHAT ARE THE BAD SUGARS (L GLUCOSE)?

If you run polarized light through L glucose or L fructose (processed sugar), the reflecting outward bends to the left. Scientists suggest that this causes the electrons to be spinning in a left ward direction. While the natural sugars, D glucose or D fructose bends the light to the right. There is conjecture that the L (left spin) decreases energy and the right hand spin increases energy. "Natural occurring sugars are D isomer. D & L sugars are mirror image of one another." (Molecular Biochemistry 1)
www.rpi.edu/dept/bebp/molbiochem/MBWeb/mb1/part2/sugar.htm

Take a look at the labels of your food to see how many sugars are in the food. If you take any breakfast cereal you will see 4 or 5 or more sugars. **L Glucose Processed Sugars**: amasake, apple sugar, **aspartame,** barbados sugar, bark sugar, barley malt, brown rice syrup, brown sugar, cane juice, cane sugar, carbitol, caramel color, concentrated fruit juice, corn syrup, date sugar, dextrin, dextrose, diglycerides, disaccharides, d-tagalose, evaporated cane juice, glycerol, glucosamine, gluconolactone, glycerides, glycerin, glycerol, glycol, hexitol, **high-fructose corn sugar (dextrose),** inverso, invert sugar, isomalt, levulose, light/lite sugar, malitol, malt dextrin, malt extract, malt syrup, malted barley, maltodextrin, maltodextrose, mannitol, mannose, maple syrup, microcrystalline cellulose, molasses, monoglycerides, monosaccarides, nectars, neotame, pentose, polydextrose, polyglycerides, powdered sugar, raisin juice/syrup, raw sugar, rice malt, rice syrup, saccyharides, sorbitol, sorghum, sugar cane, trisaccharides, turbinado sugar, unrefined sugar, white (table) sugar, xylitol, and zylose. (Source: **The Sugar Addict' Total Recovery Program,** Carolyn Dean, M.D.

L Dextrose based processed sugar destroys B Vitamins, Chromium, and Phosphorus. Processed sugar deposits in eye ducts. According to an immunologist if you eat 16+ teaspoons of sugar which equals 2 cans of soda or a couple of cookies, you will reduce the white blood cells by 92 percent and shut down the immune system for 5 hours.

DIETARY FRUCTOS OR FRUCTOSE CONTAINING SWEETENERS NEGATIVELY IMPACT OUR HEALTH

Consuming as little as 40-50 grams or slightly over 1.5 ounces of fructose over a 10 hour period may increase blood pressure, blood triglycerides, reduced insulin binding and insulin sensitivity, and increase fat weight gain. The disturbing fact is that the general population has been consuming more than that amount every day in cereals and all of our foods for the past 34 years. Total fructose consumed per person from combined consumption of sucrose and high-fructose corn syrup has increased by +26%, from 64 g/d in 1970 to 81 g/d in 1997. As Body Mass index increases (fat weight gain), the increased risk of insulin resistance, impaired glucose tolerance, hyperinsulinemia, hypertriaclglycerolemia, and hypertension may occur. (Misner, Bill)

120

121 WAYS THAT SHORT CHAINED SUGARS CAN RUIN YOUR HEALTH
(Too Much L GLUCOSE, L FRUCTOSE, and Too HIGH HEATED SUGARS)

"If glucose is present in high concentrations as free sugar, the resulting osmotic pressure could cause rupture of the cell membrane."
(http//armica.csustan.edu/principles/Lectures/03_Caron%20Coumpo unds%20in%20Cells.htm

In addition to throwing off the body's homeostasis, **excess sugar, too many short chain sugars, or the wrong kind of sugars (L-glucose & L Fructose)** may result in a number of other significant metabolic consequences: (from a variety of medical journals and other scientific publications)

1. Sugar can suppress the immune system. (Sanchez)
2. Sugar upsets the mineral relationships in the body. (Couzy)
3. Sugar can cause hyperactivity, anxiety, difficulty concentrating and crankiness in children. (Goldman)
4. Sugar can produce a significant rise in triglycerides. (Scanto)
5. Sugar contributes to the reduction in defense against bacterial infection. (Ringsdorf)
6. Sugar causes a loss of tissue elasticity and function, the more sugar you eat the more elasticity and function you lose. (Cerami)
7. Sugar reduces high density lipoproteins. (Albrink)
8. Sugar leads to chromium deficiency. (Kozlovsky)
9. Sugar leads to cancer of the breast, ovaries, prostrate, and rectum. (Takahashi)
10. Sugar can increase fasting levels of glucose. (Kelsay)
11. Sugar causes copper deficiency. (Fields)
12. Sugar can weaken eyesight and cause cataracts. (Acta Ophthalmologica) (Veromann)
13. Sugar raises the level of a neurotransmitter: domamine, serotonin, and norepinephrine. (Hence the need for Prozac) (The Addiction Letter)

14. Sugar interferes with absorption of calcium and magnesium.(Lemann)
15. Sugar can cause hypoglycemia. (Dufty)
16. Sugar can produce an over acidic digestive tract. (Dufty)
17. Sugar can cause a rapid rise of adrenaline levels in children. (Jones)
18. Sugar mal-absorbtion is frequent in patients with functional bowel disease.
19. Sugar can cause premature aging. (Lee)
20. Sugar can lead to alcoholism. (Abrahamson)
21. Sugar can cause tooth decay. (Glinsmann)
22. Sugar contributes to obesity. (Keen)
23. High intake of sugar increases the risk of Crohn's disease and ulcerative colitis.(Persson)
24. Sugar can cause changes frequently found in persons with gastric or duodenal ulcers. (Yudkin)
25. Sugar can cause arthritis. (Darlington)
26. Sugar can cause asthma. (Powers)
27. Sugar affects the growth of Candida Albicans. Long Chain sugars assist in controlling the uncontrolled growth of yeast infections). (Crook)
28. Sugar can cause gallstones. (Heaton)
29. Sugar can cause heart disease. (Yudkin)
30. Sugar can cause appendicitis. (Cleave)
31. Sugar can cause multiple sclerosis and ALS. (Erlander)
32. Sugar can cause hemorrhoids. (Cleave)
33. Sugar can elevate glucose and insulin responses in oral contraceptive users. (Behall)
34. Sugar can lead to periodontal disease. (Glinsmann)
35. Sugar can contribute to osteoporosis. (Tjaderhane)
36. Sugar contributes to saliva acidity. (Appleton)
37. Sugar can cause a decrease in insulin sensitivity and insulin resistance. (Beck)
38. Sugar can lower the amount of Vitamin E in the blood serum. (Journal of Clinical Endocrinology)
39. Sugar can cause varicose veins. (Cleave)
40. Sugar can decrease growth hormones (83). (Gardner)
41. Sugar can increase cholesterol. (Gardner)
42. Sugar can increase the systolic blood pressure. (Hodges)

43. Sugar can cause drowsiness and decreased activity in children and adults. (Behar)
44. High sugar intake increase Advanced Glycation End Products (deformed Sugars). (Furth)
45. Sugar can interfere with the absorption of protein. (Simmons)
46. Sugar can contribute to diabetes. (Diabetes)
47. Sugar can cause toxemia during pregnancy.(Cleave)
48. Sugar can contribute to eczema in children and adults. (Cleave)
49. Sugar can cause food allergies. (Appelton)
50. Sugar can cause cardiovascular diseases and atherosclerosis. (Vaccaro & Pamplona)
51. Sugar can impair the structure of DNA. (Lee)
52. Sugar can change the structure of protein. (Monnier)
53. Sugar can make our skin age by changing the structure of collagen. (Dyer)
54. Sugar and Salt can cause cataracts. (Veromann)
55. Sugar can cause emphysema. (Monnier)
56. Sugar can elevate low density lipoproteins (LDL). (Pamplona)
57. High sugar intake can impair the physiological homeostasis of many systems in the body. (Lewis)
58. Sugar lowers the enzymes ability to function. (Ceriello)
59. Sugar intake is higher in people with Parkinson's disease. (Hellenbrand)
60. Sugar can cause permanent altering in the way the proteins act in the body.
61. Sugar can increase the size of the liver by making the liver cells divide. (Goulart)
62. Sugar can increase the amount of liver fat. (Goulart)
63. Sugar can increase kidney size and produce pathological changes in the kidneys. (Yudkin)
64. Sugar can damage the pancreas. (Goulart)
65. Sugar can increase the body's fluid retention. (Goulart)
66. Sugar is enemy #1 of the bowel movement. (Goulart)
67. Sugar can cause myopia (nearsightedness). (Goulart)
68. Sugar can compromise the lining of the capillaries. (Goulart)
69. Sugar can make the tendons more brittle. (Nash)

70. Sugar can cause headaches, including migraine. (Grand)
71. Sugar plays a role in pancreatic cancer in women. (Michaud)
72. Sugar can adversely affect school children's grades and cause learning disorders. (Schauss)
73. Sugar can affect delta, alpha, and theta brain waves. (Christensen)
74. Sugar can cause depression. (Christensen)
75. Sugar can increase the risk of gastric cancer. (Cornee)
76. Sugar can cause dyspepsia (indigestion). (Yudkin)
77. Sugar can increase your risk of gout. (Yudkin)
78. Sugar can increase the levels of glucose causing indigestion of complex carbohydrates. (Riser)
79. Sugar can increase the insulin responses in humans consuming high-sugar diets compared to low sugar diets. (Riser)
80. High refined sugar diets can reduce learning capacity. (Molteni)
81. Sugar can cause less effective functioning of two blood proteins, albumin and lipoproteins, reducing the body's ability to handle fat and cholesterol.
82. Sugar can cause platelet adhesiveness. (Yudkin)
83. Sugar can contribute to Alzheimer's disease. (Frey)
84. Sugar can cause hormonal imbalance: some hormones become under active and others become overactive.(Yudkin)
85. Sugar can lead to the formation of kidney stones. (Blacklock)
86. Sugar can lead to dizziness.(Journal of Advanced Medicine. 1994; 7 (1):51-8.
87. Sugar can lead the hypothalamus to become highly sensitive to a large variety of stimuli. (Journal of Advanced Medicine)
88. Diets high in (short chain sugars) can cause free radicals and oxidative stress. (Ceriello)
89. High glucose diets can increase peripheral vascular disease.(Postgraduate medicine. Sep 1969:45:602-607
90. High sugar diet can lead to biliary tract cancer. (Lenders)
91. Sugar can feed cancer. (Moerman)

92. High sugar consumption of pregnant adolescents is associated with a two fold increased risk for delivering a small-for-gestational-age (SGA) infant. (Lenders)
93. Sugar can slow food's travel time through the gastrointestinal tract. (Kruis)
94. Sugar can increase the concentration of bile acids in stools and bacterial enzymes in the colon. (Kruis)
95. Sugar can increase estradiol (the most potent form of naturally occurring estrogen) in men. (Yudkin)
96. Sugar can combine and destroys phosphatase, an enzyme, which makes the process of digestion more difficult. (Lee)
97. Sugar can be a risk factor of gallbladder cancer. (Moerman)
98. Sugar can be an addictive substance. (Colantuoni)
99. Sugar can be intoxicating, similar to alcohol. (Colantuoni)
100. Sugar can exacerbate PMS. (The Edell Health Letter. Sep 1991; 7:1
101. Sugar given to premature babies can affect the amount of carbon dioxide they produce. (Sunehag)
102. Decrease in sugar intake can increase emotional stability. (Christensen)
103. The body changes sugar into 2 to 5 times more fat in the bloodstream than it does starch. (Nutrition Health Review. Fall 85)
104. The rapid absorption of sugar can promote excessive food intake in obese subjects. (Ludwig)
105. Sugar can worsen the symptoms of children with attention deficit hyperactivity disorder (ADHD). (Berdonces)
106. Sugar adversely affects urinary electrolyte composition. (Blacklock)
107. Sugar can slow down the ability of the adrenal glands to function. (Lechin)
108. Sugar has the potential of inducing abnormal metabolic processes in a healthy individual and promote chronic degenerative diseases. (Fields)
109. IV's (intravenous feedings) of sugar water can cut off oxygen to the brain. (Arieff)

110. High glucose intake can be an important risk factor in lung cancer. (De Stefani)
111. Sugar can increase the risk of polio. (Sandler)
112. High sugar intake can cause epileptic seizures. (Murphy)
113. Sugar can cause high blood pressure in obese people. (Stern)
114. In intensive Care Units: Limiting sugar can save lives. (Christansen)
115. Sugar may induce cell death through a Free Radical mechanism. (Donnini)
116. Sugar may impair the physiological homeostasis of body systems. (Ceriello)
117. In juvenile rehabilitation camps, when children were put on a low sugar diet, there was a 44% drop in antisocial behavior. (Schoenthaler)
118. Sugar can cause gastric cancer. (Cornee)
119. Sugar can dehydrate newborns. (Diabetes)
120. Sugar can cause gum disease.(Glinsmann)
121. Sugar can cause low birth weight babies. (Lenders)

ARE FRUCTOSE, GLUCOSE, AND SUCROSE SAFE?

There are two kinds of fructose and two kinds of glucose molecules according to www.biocheminfo.org/klotho/html/D-glucose.html. There is the natural sugar Fructose in many of the plants, fruits, and vegetables we eat. There are D Fructose and L Fructose molecules. The D Fructose and D Glucose are found in plants, while the L Fructose and L Glucose are manufactured processed sugars. When you shine polarized white light you can see the bending of the light to the left on D Fructose or D Glucose and you can see the bending of the light to the right on L Fructose (natural) or L Glucose (natural).

The same professor indicates regarding "the safety data for L glucose that its "stability is incompatible with strong oxidizing agents and has a toxicology of eye irritants." Have you ever had burning in your eyes? You are probably eating too many of the wrong kind of Sugars or too many short chain Sugars (glucose and fructose).

Many a health store or health professional touts the benefit of using Fructose sugar - a simple sugar that is made from one molecule of Glucose and 1 molecules of sucrose. Incidentally, Sucrose is made from two molecules of Glucose. Hence, Fructose is really a lot of Glucose, or 3 molecules of Glucose.

Glucose also exists in two forms, D Glucose and L Glucose. L Glucose is a natural sugar found in the body D Glucose is synthetically created in our food.

Ingestion of large quantities of fructose (and fucose) has profound metabolic consequences. It bypasses the step in glucose metabolism exerted on the rate of catabolism of glucose. This allows fructose to flood the pathways in the liver leading to enhanced fatty acid synthesis, increased esterification of fatty acids, increased VLDL, raised serum triglicerides and ultimately raising LDL concentrations, and raising uric acid leading to symptoms of gout. Also, the formations from glucose forms in the lens, the peripheral nerves, and the renal glomeruli (of the eyes) causing cataracts. Harper's Biochemistry pp. 214, 209-210.

THE PROBLEMS IN OUR DIET ARE NOT TOO MUCH FAT, BUT TOO MUCH SIMPLE SUGARS

"When the essential sugars are missing from the diet (long chain polysaccharides), the cells either cannot "talk" or they mis-communicate. The result is disease. It has been shown that dietary lack results in a defective immune response, either too much or too little. Allergic conditions are examples of an over reactive immune system. An under reactive immune system could result in an inability of the natural "killer" cells (lymphocytes) to recognize diseased cells." (Dr. Mac Robert)

The immune cells and the operation of the receptor cells are created from the good essential long chain polysaccharides.

SIMPLE SUGARS VS. COMPLEX SUGARS

A lesson can be taken from Endurance Athletes with the type of carbohydrate (sugars) used during exercise and competition. "We believe the only type any athlete should consume are long-chain (complex) carbohydrates and never short-chain carbohydrates (simple sugars). If energy products contain simple sugars (glucose, sucrose, fructose, dextrose, etc) they must be mixed in weak 6-8% solutions in order to match body fluid osmolality and be digested with any efficiency. Solutions mixed at this concentration will only provide 100 or so calories an hour, which is inadequate for maintaining energy production. Once the 6-8% solution concentration is increased osmolality is raised. Unless more water and electrolytes are added to the mix the concentrated simple sugar solution will not pass the gastric channels. Also, the athlete might very well be flirting with over hydration of his cells. If more fluids and electrolytes are not available the body will recruit these from other areas in the body to the digestive system.

"Complex sugars, however, will match body fluid osmolality with a more concentrated 15-20% solution These higher concentration complex carbohydrates (polymers) will empty the stomach at the same efficient rate as normal body fluids and provide more substantially calories (up to three times more) than simple sugar mixtures will." (Born, S)

SWEETNESS OF SUGAR

Sugar substitutes cross the blood brain barrier because of the restructuring of protein molecules to make them taste sweet.
L Fructose (not from fruit) is 166% sweeter than sucrose (table) sugar.
Neutrasweet (Aspertame) is 600% sweeter than sucrose (table) sugar.
Splenda (the newest sugar) is 900% sweeter than sucrose (table) sugar.

REFERENCES

Abrahamson, E, Peget, A, Body, Mind, and Sugar (New York: Avon, 1977.)

Albrink, M., Ullrich I H, Interaction of dietary Sucrose and Fiber on Serum Lipids in Healthy Young Men Fed High Carbohydrate Diets. American Journal of Clinical Nutrition. 1986, 43: 419-428.
128

Pamplona, R, et. Al. Mechanisma of Glycation in Atherogenesis.
Med Hypotheses, Mar 1993; 40(3); 174-81
Acta Ophthalmologica Scandinavica. Mar 2002;48;25. Taub, H Ed,
Sugar Weakens Eyesight, VM Newsletter, May 1986:06:00

Axford, John S, BS, MD, FRCP; Glycobiology & Medicine: A
Millennial Review, Lectures held at the Royal Society of Medicine,
London, UK, 11-12 July 2000

Bird, D. M.D., "Sources of Glyconutrients, the 10 Essential sugars
need in your Diet.
Australia:Hyperhealth. www.askdrbird.com/cfs/sources.htm

Born, Steve, Technical Advisor for the Health Food Industry. He is
a 3 time RAAM finisher, the 1994 Furnace Creek 508 Champion,
1999 runner-up, the only cyclist in history to complete a Double
Furnace Creek 508, and is holder of two Ultra marathon Cycling
records. In February 2004 Steve was inducted into the Ultra
Marathon Cycling Hall of Fame.

Bounous, Gustavo, McGill University, GSH, the Key to Reversing
Diseases

Bradley, David. "Cooking up Carcinogen –The chemicals generated
in our food."
New Scientist 1990, 127, issue 1729, ll Aug 1990
www.spectroscopynow.com/Spy/basehtml/SpyH/1,1181,0-5-7-0-
43571-ezine-0-5,00.html (See follow up research by Ledl)

Brown, Steve, "Amazing Sweet Magic: Diabetics Discover Sugars
that Heal," www.GlycoNutrition-Diabetes-Facts.com

Bunn, H F and Higgine P J, "Reaction of Nonosaccharides with
Proteins: Possible Evelutionary Significance," SCIENCE 213
(1961:2222-2244.

Cerami, A, Vlassara, H, Brownlee, M "Glucose and Aging."
Scientific American. May 1987:90. Lee, A, "The roles of Glycation
in Aging. Annals of the New York Academy of Science; 663:63-67.

Challem, Jack, "Is Fructose Safe,?" The Nutritional Reporter, www.wilstar.com/lowcarb/fructose.htm.

Couzy, F, et al. Behavioral effects of Sucrose (Glucose) on Preschool children. Journal of Abnormal Child Psychology. 1986:14(4):565-577.

Dills, William Jr., "Protein Fructosylation: Fructose and the Mallard Reaction,", American Journal of Clinical Nutrition 58 (1993): 779S-787S.

Dorland Medical Dictionary, http://ww.merchmedicus.com/pp/us/hcp/thepdorlands content.jsp?pg=/ppdocs/us/common/…

Fennema, OR. 1996. Food Chemistry, 3rd. Edition, Marcel Dekker, Inc, New York. Chapter 6. www.agsci.ubc.ca/courses/fnh/410/protein/1 41.htm

Foerster, A and Henie, T, "Glycation in food & metabolic transit of dietary AGEs: studies on the urinary excretion of pyraline," Institute of Food Chemistry, Technical University of Dresden, Dresden, Germany

Ganem, Bruce. "Explaining acrylamides in food – how acrylamide formed when starch-rich foods are fried or baked," Journal of Chemical and Engineering News, Dec 2, 2002, www.innovations-report.com/html/reports/life_sciences/report-15409.html

Gugliucci, Dr. A., "The Sour Side of Sugar, Why do crust pies, cola drinks, coffee, ice cream and your body protein cause you to suffer from diabetes." http//209.209.34.25/webdocs/Glycation%20Page/Glycation%20Page.htm

Harper's Biochemistry, GlycoProteins, Chapter 56, 1996 Edition Mirkin, Gabe M.D., "Acrylamide, a class of chemicals that form advanced glycation end products," www.drmirkin.com/nutrition/1220.html.

Halifrisch, J, et al., "The effects of fructose on Blood Lipid Levels," American Journal of Clinical Nutrition 37, no, 3 (1983): 740-748

Hollenbeck, Clair B, "Dietary Fructose Effects on Lipoprotein Metabolism and Risk for Coronary Artery Disease," American Journal of Clinical Nutrition 58 (1993): 800S-807S

Ledl, Franze, Schleicher, Erwin. Stutgart University. Academic Hospital of Munich-Schwaging (W. Germany). Reported in Angew. Chem. Int. Edn. England 1990, 29, 565.
Life Extension Research, "Glycation Role in Inflammation," www.lifeextensionvitamins.com/chinpa2.html

Lyons, David, "Telomere research reveals intriguing paradox," Dept of Energy's Los Alamos, E.O. Berkeley National Laboratories, Sloan-Kettering Cancer Center, 505 665 9298, www.lanl.gov/worldview/news/releases/archive/00-057.shtml

Dr. Iain MacRobert FRACA FCOohthHKam: An Open Letter to Mankind, www.glycohealthservice.com/s-macrobert openletter.htm

O"Brien, John, Nursten, Harry, Crabbe, M.J.D., Ames, Jennifer; "The Maillard Reaction in Food Medicine (Chemical reactions in chemistry, food science, medicine, carcinogen in foods, health, and disease), 464 pages, $197.00.

Rumessen, J J and Gudmand-Hoyer, "Functional Bowel Disease; Malabsorbtion and Abdominal Distress after ingestion of Fructose, Sorbitol, and Fructose-Sorbitol Mixtures," Gastroenterology 95 no. 3, (September 1988): 694-700.

Scopes, RK. 1994. Protein Purification: Principles and Practice. 3rd. Edition. Springer-Verlag, New York, Inc. P. 95-101.

Somersall, Allan C. Ph.D., M.D>, "Breakthrough in Cell-Defense,"

Somersall, Allan C. Ph.D., M.D>, "Nature's Goldmine- Harvesting Miracle Ingredients from MILK."

Spiegel, Allen M. M.D., "G Proteins, Receptors, and Disease –
Contemporary Endocrinology, Chief, metabolic Diseases Branch,
National Institute of Diabetes and Digestive and Kidney Disease,
National Institutes of Health."

University of Victory, Canada, Biochemistry 300,
http://web.uvic.ca/biochem/courses/bioc300/NutrBioc300.htm

Wautier, J.L., Guillausseau, P.J., "Advanced Glycation End
Products (AGE), their Receptors & Diabetic Angiopathy,"

Zakim, D and Herman, R H, "Fructose metabolism II," American
Journal of Clinical Nutrition 21:315-319. 1958

SECTION THREE
CHAPTER ONE
MENTAL HAS A PROFOUND INFLUENCE ON PHYSICAL

Some people love to get attention any way they can. One woman was starting to feel marvelous after using a product and decided to stop taking it because to quote her "My husband pays more attention to me when I am not feeling well." She suffered with arthritis because her need for attention from her husband was greater than her need for good health.

We encounter people who consistently talk of their health woes. It's so much a part of their life that it is the only reference point they have.

I also know people who have much to complain about yet they are accomplishing so much in their life. Chris, a quadriplegic got his Eagle Scout. He gave instruction to others how to accomplish each particular merit badge. His art was drawn by his mouth. It was truly awe inspiring. A book was written about him called "The Flight of the Crippled Eagle" by Donna Marie Shaffer.

I love the Olympics. All the skills the athletes perfect, are inspiring. I have a special admiration for the Special Olympics and the people who work with them.

They are operating in their excellence. Attention is good. It makes a person feel people care. Talking about how sick we are sends off negative energy while the energy we get while we are accomplishing something great is positive.

If a person comes to me with their concerns and I can see that they want to shift to a successful positive place, I don't mind hearing them out; but as for those who make excuses and blame every one else, I'll either not listen or I'll give them feedback.

I have lived my life trying to keep everyone else out of pain's way. I grieved for those who were in poverty, for those who were lame in spirit and body, for those who were grimy, smelly or offensive; for those who were unattractively to thin or too huge.

I finished being angry with those persons who have done things that cause me to grieve realizing that everyone does pretty much what they know how to do. And often they do what they do because they deeply love and are tying to save a person from pain when they actually do what causes the most pain.

I have said I was sorry so many times in the past, people thought I was guilty. I was only sorry for their pain, not that I had caused it or could have done any differently.

I take a look at what causes me so much pain because I realize there are times that a person can hurt because of self absorbed pity. Because of the great amount of persecution that I have received in many forms, I have learned to look at the good things around me and pretty much ignore the uncomfortable.

I have learned how to keep it from destroying me physically. Will I give up what it takes to overcome pain or do other things to keep me healthy? If not, I have signed my own Death Certificate..

If there is anyone who detests another or blames another for anything, I invite you to take a look at yourself to see if you are not the cause of your own pain.

When we have a great desire for something, we need to give something else up for it. But never give anything up for something else when you are angry or miserable. It will be for the wrong reason. And it may be the wrong thing to give up.

Some possibilities

:Great Desire	Give Up	Do instead
1. Home	Vices	Barter
2. Car	Shopping	Shop Thrift shops
3. Boat	Malls	Do it yourself
4. Vacation	Beauty	Give up your ego
5. Baby	Treatments	Live simple 'til you get your
6. Health	Dining out	desire
7. Wealth	Your ego	Be patient and enjoy the
8. Peace &	Greed	journey
Harmony	Selfishness	Network yourself in service
	Doubt	Layers of Light
		www.2lolii.com/dandyone

MONEY WE SPEND

Addictions can be caused by either mental or physical problems or both. We spend money and it is often spent on some lust or craving such as the detrimental sugars, detrimental fats and vices.

Our health is an investment for now and for our future. Sometimes it is an investment of time and sometimes it's of money. The thoughts we entertain and the books we read are an investment in time. The service we perform is also an investment in time. Our thoughts invested now create what we will have in the future.

Someone once said , "I don't criticize because when I do, I get it."

At the high school I went to, I tried out for A Cappella Choir. I got in. We traveled the state of California competing. We were the best. Our scores were A-1 always. There were ten of us who were the best of the best. We were good and I knew it. We toured the state of California in 1960 and 1961. There were three sopranos, three Altos, two tenors and two basses. I was first Alto.

I didn't enjoy music much unless I was singing it. I was annoyed by terrible singers. Then I got it. I got so ill with no energy that I could sing no longer. I criticized and I got it. At Impact Training I learned to enjoy music and it touched my soul. I got cured from criticizing.

Just a few thoughts

A little girl was completely tone deaf. She sang in the car and her brothers insulted her. They were told to leave her alone and that it was ok. She practiced and practiced and practiced. She practiced so much that she was accepted into an elite group of girls that sang and danced and traveled to different parts of the world. The talent will come if you keep persisting

A man had children who seemed to be always depressed. He didn't understand them at all. It was quite hard to deal with. Then he was uprooted from friends and everything familiar and he learned how it felt to be depressed. Experience teaches compassion

A man never had a health problem. He didn't understand anyone being ill. When he got ill, he became more understanding

If you don't understand someone's apparent follies, don't judge or maybe you will get it so you can understand.

There are things to do to inspire and humble you without having to go through unfortunate experiences: read, read and read.

Your words give you away. Before you speak, realize that what you say will remain in the minds of the other person long after you do not feel that way any more.

It is because light travels faster than sound, some people appear to be bright until they speak.

If you are going to think it and say something about it, you may be surprised at the wisdom you will gain by what the other person says in response.

Learn when to speak and when to hold back. Learn to speak without accusations. Example: I feel this way when you say that, instead of you made me feel this way. No one makes you feel. You do that on your own.

A SMILE

A smile costs nothing, but gives much.
It enriches those who receive,
without making poorer those who give.
It takes but a moment,
but the memory of it sometimes lasts forever.

None is so rich or mighty
that he can get along without it,
and none is so poor
that he cannot be made rich by it.
A smile creates happiness in the home,
Fosters good will in business
And is the countersign of friendship.

It brings rest to the weary,
cheer to the discouraged, sunshine to the sad,
and it is nature's best antidote for trouble.
Yet it cannot be bought, begged, borrowed or stolen,
for it is something that is of no value to anyone
until it is given away.

Some people are too tired to give you a smile.
Give them one of yours,
As none needs a smile so much
As he who has no more to give.

The Circle of Giving and Receiving

Many of us have heard the expression "Giving is its own reward", and while this statement is certainly true, and is more than reason enough to give, there's another aspect of giving that many fail to recognize. Giving is an energy that not only helps others but creates even more for the person who is doing the giving. This is a natural law that is true regardless of whether the person who is giving wants or even realizes what is occurring.

Money is "circulation." It needs to flow. When you are frightened, selfish, or when you hoard everything for yourself, you literally stop the circulation. You create "clogged pipes," making it difficult to

137

keep money flowing back in your direction. Any success you have is despite your lack of giving, not because of it. The way to get the flow going again is to start giving. Be generous. Pay others well, tip your waitress that extra dollar. Support several charities. Give back. Watch what happens! Things will start popping up out of nowhere.

The same dynamic is true if you want to fill your life with love or anything else worthwhile. Giving and receiving are two sides of the same coin. If you want more love, or fun, or respect, or success, or anything else, the way to get it is simple: give it away: Don't worry about a thing. The universe knows what it's doing. Everything you give away will return, with interest.

There is a scripture that states, "Cast your bread upon the waters and in many days it will return." I like to add "buttered."

Sometimes it is necessary to do what we feel right about even when it isn't customary. When we do risk, we often create great value. Here is a story about a mother who risked and the value was great. The story is public domain but the names are changed.

A gift to give/determined commitment

When Ellen found out that another baby was on the way, she helped her 3-year old son, Tony, prepare for a new sibling. They found out that the new baby was going to be a girl, and day after day, night after night, Tony sang to his sister in Mommy's tummy.

The pregnancy progressed normally for Ellen. Then the labor pains came. Every five minutes: Every minute. But complications arose during delivery and hours of labor. Finally, Tony's little sister was born but she was in serious condition. The baby was rushed by ambulance to a neonatal intensive care unit at another hospital.

Days went by. The little girl got worse. The pediatric specialist told the parents, "There is very little hope. Be prepared for the worst." Ellen and her husband contacted a local cemetery about a burial plot. They had fixed up a special room in their home for the new baby, now they planned a funeral. Tony kept begging his parents to let him see his sister, "I want to sing to her," he said.

After two weeks it looked like a funeral would come before the end of the week. Tony kept nagging about singing to his sister, but kids are never allowed in Intensive Care. But Ellen made up her mind. She decided to take Tony whether they liked it or not. If he couldn't see his sister then, he may never see her alive.

She dressed him in an oversized scrub suit and marched him into ICU. He looked like a walking laundry basket, but the head nurse recognized him as a child and bellowed, "Get that kid out of here now! No children are allowed in ICU."

The mother rose up strong in Ellen, and the usually mild mannered lady glared steel-eyed into the head nurse's face, her lips a firm line. "He is not leaving until he sings to his sister!"

Ellen got Tony to his sister's bedside. He gazed at the tiny infant losing the battle to live. In the pure hearted voice of a 3 year old, Tony sang: "You are my sunshine, my only sunshine, you make me happy when skies are gray—"Instantly the baby girl responded. The pulse rate became calm and steady.

Tony kept singing, "You never know, dear, how much I love you, Please don't take my sunshine away---" The ragged, strained breathing become as smooth as a kitten's purr.

Tony kept singing "The other night, dear, as I lay sleeping, I dreamed I held you in my arms." Tony's little sister relaxed as rest, healing rest, swept over her.

Tears welled up in the eyes of the bossy head nurse, Ellen glowed. "You are my sunshine, my only sunshine. Please don't take my sunshine away."

Perception

There is a saying that one man's junk is another man's treasure. There are some things that have special meaning to one person while the other person finds no value in it. This story gives an example.

Positive thoughts - Positive actions - Positive results

One day an eight year old boy went to the pet store with his dad to buy a puppy. The store manager showed them to a pen where five little furry balls huddled together.

After a while, the boy noticed one of the litter all by itself in an adjacent pen.

The boy asked, "Why is that puppy all alone?"

The manager explained, the puppy was born with a bad leg and would be crippled for life, so we're going to have to put him to sleep."

"You're going to kill this little puppy?" the boy said sadly while patting it.

"You have to realize that this puppy would never be able to run and play with a boy like you."

"After a short conversation with his boy, the dad told the manager that they wanted to buy the puppy with the bad leg.

"For the same amount of money, you could have one of the 'healthy' ones. Why do you want this one?"

To answer the manager's question, the boy bent over and pulled up the pants on his right leg, exposed the brace underneath and said, "Mister, I want this one because I understand what he's going through.

In this next story, this man's perception is that "It's all good." I love that expression. It is usually the positive individuals who use it.

The names have been changed

140

Positive thoughts - Positive actions - Positive results

Your attitude is your choice

Larry is the kind of guy you love to hate. He is always in a good mood and always has something positive to say. When someone would ask him how he was doing, he would reply, "If I were any better, I would be twins."

He was a unique manager because he had several waiters who had followed him around from restaurant to restaurant. The reason the waiters followed Larry was because of his attitude. He was a natural motivator.

If an employee was having a bad day, Larry was there telling the employee how to look on the positive side of the situation. Seeing this style really made me curious, so one day I went to Larry and asked him, "I don't get it! You can't be a positive person all of the time. How do you do it?" Larry replied, "Each morning I wake up and say to myself, Larry, you have two choices today. You can choose to be in a good mood or you can choose to be in a bad mood. I choose to be in a good mood. Each time something bad happens, I can choose to be a victim or I can choose to learn from it. I choose to learn from it. Every time someone comes to me complaining, I can choose to accept their complaining or I can point out the positive side of life. I choose the positive side of life

Life is all about choices. When you cut away all the junk, every situation is a choice. You choose how you react to situations. You choose how people will affect your mood. You choose to be in a good mood or bad mood. The bottom line: It's your choice how you live life."

I reflected on what Larry said. Soon thereafter, I left the restaurant industry to start my own business. We lost touch, but I often thought about him when I made a choice about life instead of reacting to it.

Several years later, I heard that Larry did something you are never supposed to do in a restaurant business: he left the back door open

141

one morning and was held up at gun point by three armed robbers. While trying to open the safe, his hand, shaking from nervousness, slipped off the combination. The robbers panicked and shot him. Luckily, Larry was found relatively quickly and rushed to the local trauma center.

After 18 hours of surgery and weeks of intensive care, Larry was released from the hospital with fragments of the bullets still in his body.

I saw Larry about six months after the accident. When I asked him how he was, he replied, "If I were any better, I'd be twins. Wanna see my scars?"

I declined to see his wounds, but did ask him what had gone through his mind as the robbery took place. "The first thing that went through my mind was that I should have locked the back door. Then, as I lay on the floor, I remembered that I had two choices: I could choose to live or I could choose to die. I chose to live."

"The paramedics were great. They kept telling me I was going to be fine. But when they wheeled me into the ER and I saw the expressions on the faces of the doctors and nurses, I got really scared."

"In their eyes, I read 'he's a dead man." I knew I needed to take action. There was a big burly nurse shouting questions at me. She asked if I was allergic to anything. 'Yes' I replied. The doctors and nurses stopped working as they waited for my reply. I took a deep breath and yelled, 'Bullets!' Over their laughter, I told them, 'I am choosing to live. Operate on me as if I am alive, not dead."

As a man thinketh so is he. He lived because he decided to live.

Positive thoughts - Positive actions - Positive results

Unconditional love

This story is about a woman who was a very friendly person and always smiled at everyone and said hello. so when the class was given an assignment by the teacher to go out and smile at three people and document the reactions, she thought it would be a piece of cake literally. One crisp March morning, soon after the project was assigned, she, her husband and youngest son went out to McDonald's. It was just their way of sharing special play time with their son. They were standing in line, waiting to be served, when all of a sudden everyone around them began to back away, including her husband. The woman did not move an inch. An overwhelming feeling of panic welled up inside of her as she turned to see why they had moved.

As the woman turned around she smelled a horrible "dirty body" smell and standing behind her were two poor homeless men. As she looked down at the short gentleman, he was smiling. His beautiful sky blue eyes were full of God's Light as he searched for acceptance. He said, 'Good day' as he counted the few coins he had been clutching. The second man fumbled with his hands as he stood behind his friend. The woman realized the second man was mentally deficient and the blue eyed gentleman was his salvation. She held back tears as she stood there with them. The young lady at the counter asked him what they wanted. He said "coffee is all Miss." They had to buy something to be able to sit in the restaurant and that is all they could afford. They just wanted to be warm. The woman felt a compulsion that was so great she almost reached out and embraced the little man with the blue eyes. That is when she noticed all eyes in the restaurant were set on her. She felt like they were judging her every action.

The woman smiled and asked the young lady behind the counter to give her two more breakfast meals on a separate tray. She then walked around the corner to the table the men had chosen as a resting spot. She put the tray on the table and laid her hand on the blue eyed gentlemen's cold hand. He looked up at her with tears in his eyes and said "Thank you." She leaned over, began to pat his hand and said "I did not do this for you. God is here working through me to give you hope." She started to cry as she walked away to join her husband and son.

Positive thoughts - Positive actions - Positive results

The Old Mule

This parable is told of a farmer who owned an old mule. The mule fell into the farmer's well. The farmer heard the mule 'braying' or whatever mules do when they fall into wells. After carefully assessing the situation, the farmer sympathized with the mule but decided that neither the mule nor the well was worth the trouble of saving. Instead, he called his neighbors together, told them what had happened. . . and enlisted them to help haul dirt to bury the old mule in the well and put him out of his misery.

Initially, the old mule was hysterical! But as the farmer and his neighbors continued shoveling and the dirt hit his back . . . a thought struck him. It suddenly dawned on him that every time a shovel load of dirt landed on his back ... HE WOULD SHAKE IT OFF AND STEP UP! This he did, blow after blow. "Shake it off and step up . . . shake it off and step up . . . shake it off and step up!" he repeated to encourage himself. No matter how painful the blows, or how distressing the situation seemed, the old mule fought "panic" and just kept right on SHAKING IT OFF AND STEPPING UP!

It wasn't long before the old mule, battered and exhausted, stepped triumphantly over the wall of that well. What seemed like it would bury him actually helped him . . . all because of the manner in which he handled his adversity. THAT'S LIFE. If we face our problems and respond to them positively, and refuse to give in to panic, bitterness, or self-pity, the adversities that come along to bury us, usually have within them the very real potential to benefit us!

Never be afraid to try something new. Remember that amateurs built the ark . . . . Professionals built the Titanic.

Positive-thoughts-Positive actions-Positive results

On the other hand, negative thoughts can canker us as in the next story.

144

Perception: Judgment.

A Young man was getting ready to graduate from college. For many months he had admired a beautiful sports car in a dealer's showroom, and knowing his father could well afford it, he told him that was all he wanted. As Graduation Day approached, the young man awaited signs that his father had purchased the car. Finally, on the morning of his graduation, his father called him into his private study. His father told him how proud he was to have such a fine son and told him how much he loved him. He handed his son a beautifully wrapped gift box. Curious and somewhat disappointed, the young man opened the box and found a lovely, leather-bound Bible, with the young man's name embossed in gold. Angry, he raised his voice to his father and said, "with all your money, you give me a Bible? ...And stormed out of the house.

Many years passed and the young man was very successful in business. He had a beautiful home and wonderful family, but realized his father was very old and thought perhaps he should go to him. He had not seen him since that graduation day. Before he could make arrangements, he received a telegram telling him his father had passed away, and willed all of his possessions to his son. He needed to come home immediately and take care of things. When he arrived at his father's house, sudden sadness and regret filled his heart. He began to search through his father's important papers and saw the still new Bible, just as he had left it years ago. With tears, he opened the Bible and began to turn the pages. His father had carefully underlined a verse, Matt. 7-11, "And if ye, being evil, know how to give good gifts to your children, how much more shall your Heavenly Father which is in Heaven, give to those who ask Him?"

As he read those words, a car key dropped from the back of the Bible. It had a tag with the dealer's name, the same dealer who had the sports car he had desired. On the tag was the date of his graduation, and the words PAID IN FULL.

Positive Thought - Positive Action - Positive results.
Even when it doesn't seem like it in the beginning

Years ago, I assumed that my husband could do something or other. He got really irritated with me. I couldn't figure out why he got so upset. In his mind was I mocking his inability to do it? Was he being stubborn because he didn't want to do it for me? Maybe I wasn't worth it. Maybe he just didn't think he could do it and I was pestering him to do something that he knew he could not do. My faith in him resulted in unpleasantness but I continued to have faith in him and he started doing things that he didn't even think he could do and was so impressed with his projects.

Perceptions are mere beliefs that feel real and honest. Perceptions are real. They should not be discounted. They will stay real until the person has more input to release or change perception and then a new perception is acquired. There is a saying "The more a person knows, the more the person realizes the less the person knows. We sometimes make judgments from our perceptions. It is important that we are careful in what we judge.

Judgments

There is a scripture that states "Judge not that ye be not judged." There are two forms of judging. One is condemnatory and the other is choice making. We are required to condemn no man. To judge with the purest sense is extremely beneficial. I have the right to judge or make a decision whether I do this or that, whether I say this or that. It is called a matter of choice.

So doesn't that mean the following?

Judge = condemn: doesn't work. Too much negative energy
Judge = make a choice: does work. But then let it go. It takes too much energy think about why I made the choice and what might happen if I made a different one.

Judging can be an energy drain. People who are in that line of work are getting paid for it so there is an exchange: Some sort of compensation for the action. If you are in that line of work, I'm sure that you regain that energy by doing something fun, relaxing or rejuvenating.

It can be life altering to judge or not to judge an act or action. Make your character judgment ahead of time and stick with it so that when you are in that moment you will not be confused. The jails and prisons are full of people who got caught up in things because they

146

didn't commit themselves to making choices and when the time came they committed themselves to another person or people who led them into tragedy.

Even when heathenish things are done, it is not our right to judge that person. If we spend our time loving and consoling the grieving, our temporarily spent energy will be revived again.

Without judgment, no energy is spent: just peace and joy

Scenario

Thanksgiving dinner with cousins, aunts, uncles, brother, sisters, moms and dads: "I don't want to go in the kitchen to help because it's too dirty in there" or "I would help but the kitchen is too dirty."

In these statements we learn: The kitchen is dirty. The guest doesn't want to help.

If you were one of the guests could you have found yourself in judgment? There was nothing wrong with her choice, but if there had been condemnation, it would have been an energy drain. I'm not even going to go into any possible condemnation. It does not work.

Let's instead take a look at the rest of the story. There is always something more.

The Host:
Traditionally thanksgiving had been at another family members' home, but she couldn't have it this year so another sister offered to have it at her house even though there was not much time to prepare. She appeared worried that her performance as a host was not good enough. She made apologies and gave reasons for this or for that until she recognized that everyone was having a wonderful time. She had a full time job with active teens, sub-teens and friends. She hadn't been on the job long and it was extremely stressful. She was involved with youth outside the home as well, and involved with the building of her new home. The two boys spent time in the orchards working with Dad who all came home to eat for lunch and return to

147

the orchards. Even some of the cousins ventured out to see the orchard. They could have chosen to not have thanksgiving dinner there and break tradition. Instead of judging, the family went about assisting and visiting and in no time all was taken care of. There was not another thought about the condition of the kitchen. People spend so much time worrying about something or trying to figure it out or figure out if it is right or wrong or good or bad, they forget to enjoy life and it's experiences. They forget to have compassion and give up a part of freedom.

The Guest
At home the guest has three children of her own: two in diapers, one in school. She is Room Mother, helps out each week at school and makes and sells crafts to help with income. Her husband bought her a sewing machine and told her to earn it. She paid him back for it by making things and selling them. She sings at various functions, spends time practicing because though she has an incredibly beautiful voice she needs a lot of practice. Children come over to play, she cooks from scratch, the only way her husband will allow. Her kitchen is always clean even when she has extremely hard pregnancies. She doesn't have much help from hubby during this particular time because he's very sought after in the business world and community work. He was cheery, optimistic and never sick. He has no idea what it's like and says sickness is in the mind. Although there is some truth to that, it doesn't help to be reminded of it when you are suffering. He changed his thinking a little when his mother died of cancer but that was cancer. The guest was a sickly child, born early and had near death experiences and persecution galore. There was constant vigilance on her mothers' part to keep her alive. It was she who made the statement about not helping because the kitchen was dirty. Not a week earlier she came close to a nervous breakdown. She sang a song and asked her husband if it sounded good. He said. "It'd sound better if you'd practice." He seldom praised her: just expected so much that she couldn't perform any more so she experienced an acute panic attack.

The real reason she didn't want to help in the kitchen was because she was so ill, which became evident as the day wore on. She might have been thinking "I feel so ill right now and I'm embarrassed to be ill, but I feel guilty not helping, so I'll make a different excuse."
148

There are so many variables in life that it is such a waste of time to judge another.

Later that day the guest collapsed. The body collapses when it can take no more. Requiring attention is sometimes a way of survival. Survival mechanisms show up in many ways. Can we turn our head or ignore it and be less compassionate because it doesn't look proper?

Both Host and Guest needed attention. People stepped in and assisted the Host with the duties of the kitchen and dinner and others stepped in to assist the guest in her need for assistance. Everything turned out simply wonderfully. The food was exceptional and the company was equally great.

There is something to be said about the attention we give to other people. If we overact our concerns by doting or even thinking "look at me, I'm helping", we are being artificial. You don't have to over act for people to know you are concerned. You also do not have to under act, thinking if you show too much concern the person will keep it up and take advantage.

When concern is given without over acting or under acting, people usually heal much faster. They got what they needed and are ready to get on with life on their own. When they don't get what they need, it is called need deficiency, or need deprivation. There are a lot of deficiencies or deprivations that are damaging: Some are
1.　　Love deficiency:
2.　　Nutrient deficiency:
3.　　Touch deficiency: Many years ago I went to visit a baby in a Hospital in New York City. He had a growth on his forehead. I walked by crib after crib noticing that the babies seemed lethargic and really not interested in anything around them. They were literally abandoned babies that lie there with touch from no one. The nurses were busy and that's just the way it was. The babies had no visitors. With no touch the baby refused to eat and if a baby was not wanted on the outside they were left to

die. It was heart wrenching. Many people want to adopt and the system does not make it easy to do so.

4. Attention deficiency: Interaction is a vital part of growing up emotionally healthy. If a person is attention deficit, he/she will tend to zone out and be unaware of the surroundings. Learning life's lessons are not as readily available to them. They can immerse themselves in books and if the books are beneficial, this can be a great benefit. If the material they are reading is counter productive, it can be even dangerous.

5. Need Deficiency: Although some people refuse to acknowledge need and claim "They Deserve it" we have many needs. We do deserve things that are for our good. While we have definite needs, it is important that we go for our needs and desires. Need efficiency causes one to be withdrawn and feel abandoned.

There are a couple of my favorite stories about not judging because, you never know.

Maybe so; maybe not

Once in a village far away there lived a wise man. One day a farmer came to the wise man and said, "Oh wise man, the most terrible thing has happened to me. My ox has died and I have no way to plant my crop and will not be able to feed my family and we will die. Isn't this the worst thing that could happen to me? "Maybe so; maybe not," said the wise man. The farmer left the wise man and stormed into the village declaring to everyone that the wise man had gone crazy. The next day or so the farmer was in his field and a horse wandered by. The farmer caught the horse and was able to get a lot more done. He went to the wise man and said, "Oh wise man, you were right. It is a good thing that my ox died. I never would have bothered to catch that horse and I would never have been able to get my crops in so fast. The wise man replied again "Maybe so; maybe not." Now the farmer went into the village and proclaimed that the wise man had really lost it now. A few days later the farmer's son fell off the horse and broke his leg. The farmer hurried back to the wise man and cried "Oh wise man, you were right. It was not good that the ox died and I got the horse 'cause my son has fallen off the horse and broken his leg. Once again the wise man

150

only said "Maybe so; maybe not." Now the farmer was really infuriated. This wise man had gone mad and once again he went to the village to tell the people. A few days later a war broke out and all the young men from the village went to war and were all killed except for the farmer's son who had a broken leg.

Not always what it seems

A young man wished to purchase a gift for his new sweetheart's birthday, and as they had not been dating very long, after careful consideration, decided a pair of gloves would strike the right note: romantic but not too personal.

Accompanied by his sweetheart's younger sister, he went to a department store and bought a pair of white gloves. The younger sister purchased a pair of panties for herself. During the wrapping, the clerk mixed up the items and the sister got the gloves and the sweetheart got the panties. Without checking the contents, he sealed the package and mailed it to the sweetheart with this note: Darling, I chose these because I noticed that you are not in the habit of wearing any when we go out in the evening: If it had not been for your sister, I would have chosen the long ones with the buttons, but she wears the short ones that are easy to remove.

These are a delicate shade, but the lady I bought them from showed me the pair she had been wearing for the past three weeks and they were hardly soiled. I had her try yours on for me and she looked really smart.

I wish I was there to put them on you for the first time, as no doubt other hands will come in contact with them before I have a chance to see you again.

When you take them off, remember to blow in them before putting them away as they will naturally be a little damp from wearing.

Just think how many times I will kiss them during the coming year. I hope you will wear them for me on Friday night. The latest style is to wear them folded down with a little fur showing. All My Love.

One can make a difference.

One day a young male teen shoveled the snow off an elderly women's walkway and left before she knew who it was that had done such a kind deed. When the woman saw what was done for her, she could think of five people who might have done this and went to her kitchen and made five pies. She delivered them to their houses and left before they knew who did it. When each of the people opened their five doors and saw the pies on their porch, they got busy and did a kind deed for other people who they thought might have done this kind deed. It takes less than 30 days to fill the world and it often comes back to you.

See the movie "Pay it forward."

Let's make sure we do not make a difference in the reverse way. It could end up coming back to you and cause a big upheaval. Let's be careful how we act on the freeway when someone cuts in front of us. (blank) is already having a bad day and

1.   You flip him off. He goes home and yells at his wife. She sends the kids out in anger, the kids hit a dog or cat. The cat dashes off and gets hit by a car. It happens to be your favorite pet and you killed him. Or, yell at the wife who spanks the kid who drowns the cat or hits a kid at school who goes home and damages his dad's boat. The boat that you were going fishing in. The dad didn't notice the leak so you and he go fishing and when you were in the middle of the lake. You started sinking, Your vicious actions always return to haunt you.

2.   You smile and wave him on. He goes home and hugs his wife. The family gets together for an activity. Your favorite pet gets lost and wanders by the family. They make arrangements to find the owner of the pet and you drive by and notice a sign saying "dog found." It is your dog. Your goods deeds always come back to bless you.

3.   Of course these are short versions of what could really happen but you get the picture. It is called the ripple effect. In the scriptures, it is the same as saying "Cast

your bread upon the waters and in many days it will be returned" (buttered).

Don't stress if you slip up here and there. Just make every effort to do the best you can to send out positives as often as you have an opportunity.

Sometimes we make decisions that we know might hurt us in the short run but are projecting success in the long run.

We are creating with everything we think, say and do. If it doesn't go the way we hoped for, it is still a choice that we made and we should not regret the freedom of our choices.

The next story is based on true facts, the names have been changed and there has been a huge change that took place in the people involved.

I need to express the need to not judge. A head injury can cause people to do and be who they are not. The brain goes through processes that the injured person has to adjust to and it takes many years. Healing is accelerated by excellent therapists and understanding parents. It is necessary to use different ways to work with a person who has had head injuries. There is a way. There is always a way. Sometimes things are seemingly hopeless but turn out to be a blessing.

The trial of this family would have been insurmountable without patience and commitment to the cause of helping a son. The patience is paying off.

"Carol's husband had, for a long time, wanted to open a store. When he was dismissed from his job, they took it fairly well in spite of the circumstances, and proclaimed, "When one door closes, another one opens." They decided to make it a family business where everyone could participate. Two of the children wanted to help but one was driven out by the other. They had already invested over $100,000.00, plus a mortgage. They needed to make it work. It was much harder than they expected.

Carol and Mike had picked Dean up from another state in the late fall of 1999. He was living in a drug and crime infested neighborhood where a few people had been killed. He was comfortable enough there but they were concerned about his safety and hoped that by bringing him out of that environment, he would make changes in his life. He basically lived multiple lives after he arrived at his parent's home. He was one person to his parents, another person to his girl friend and so forth. He had had a problem with drugs and alcohol, but was making some real improvement when he got into a truck/motorcycle accident. He was on his way from one job to another when a truck pulled out in front of him. His pelvis was separated, he had a cracked scull that resulted in brain trauma and his good leg was broken and twisted. A few years earlier, he was caught up in a net and drug from the back of a pick up truck which resulted in numerous injuries including his head, leg and foot which never healed completely. This resulted in, both legs being damaged.

Dean was given drugs in the hospital and his addiction returned. He went through another period of pain medication and alcohol to ward off the pain. It wasn't illegal to drink or take prescription drugs so he pretty much got away with the addiction except for a few bouts in the ambulance and hospital.

It was a year after this that Carol and Mike opened their store. Soon after they opened, Dean came to assist and his friends started frequenting the store. Carol kept a pretty close watch on them but she wasn't there all of the time. She saw them sneak off at times. Within the year, three of his friends died of an overdose. It woke him up some. He had a family now and was keeping busy. He was
154

receiving counseling and was starting to do really well but there were setbacks that proved to be extremely painful and stressful for the family.

There were some of those humiliating instances and financial losses that come along with drug abuse and head trauma but his parents would not give up. Dean was doing the best he could but it still did not seem enough to make a real difference.

During this year Mike had many repairs and some major renovations on the properties co owned by his parents and brother including the one Dean lived in. Often Dean was left alone to run the store. Dean loved the flea market and pawn shop mentality. With Dean there it started to look like a pawn shop having acquired more things than was denoted in the store name. Some of the displays were not professional looking and people asked if it was a pawn shop. Carol told people "no. But we buy, sell, trade so it looks a little like one." The stigmatism remained. Sales plummeted but by the time that happened, their debt had diminished. Dean would not listen to Carol and did things his way. There were some ways in which he helped but the mistakes were costly. He cared about his parents so much but didn't trust that they could run the store on their own, so when Carol told him what needed to be done he wouldn't listen.

During the first year he had run people off and had the city and neighborhood intent on shutting them down. There were a number of people however, that really loved him. They were people from AA, the jail or down and outers. Dean loved to buy, sell and trade. He often bought when there were bills to pay. He thought all that was needed was $3000.00 to keep their doors open and when that happened, he was ready to stash the cash: not always for his own gain but he bought things for the store that were not wanted. In reality, the cost to run the business was more like $9500.00 without taking a draw. Carol was putting all her money from her job into the business and charging money to a son's credit card. She could not go back to work because of illness and all her retirement went to personal and business expenses. Dean had to do about four months in jail. He was able to get on work release because of Carol's illness and his parents' need for his assistance. They could have decided right then, "Here is our chance to get someone else in here and train them," but it was a family business and Dean had shown such progress, they decided that even though he had no license to drive, they'd pick him up and drop him off when his wife couldn't do it. Carol arranged with Deans wife to pick him up and Carol or Mike could get him back. Arrangements were made but Sara refused to assist. Once in a while Dean got rides. He did pretty well. If he hadn't, Carol would have abolished the arrangement. When he got out of jail, there wasn't as much pressure to do so well

Dean seemed to remember all the money he put in the till but never kept track of what he took out. There were times he kept the money aside so he could give his Dad money to buy things. He saw how happy it made his Dad feel.

The issue was not that he took money out of the business. He did help out. Dean acted like or seemed to think he put more money in the business than he took out. The issue was, "Do not buy junk that we can not sell." The situation ultimately helped the impoverished community. Mike started giving merchandise to people who were in need. Some of them were in and out of jail, drug addicts and people with mental imbalances. Mike helped many. Some came back to bite him and others are dear good people.

If "he is the store," as his counselors have surmised, he stole it. In order for Dean to get his way, he screamed and threatened. He drove his sibling out of the store and later drove Carol out He had people believing that he was the only one helping and other family members were good for nothing. Dean acknowledged that they were the way they were because of his behavior toward them when he was younger; yet he was angry because they did not respond to him; his fear tactics with them did not get the results he wanted. They helped in other ways and they caused little or no stress. Dean was Carol's biggest stressor. She was committed to being healthy and stress was not helping. The poem "The Desiderata" was apropos and Carol made every effort to follow that as she could. "Avoid loud and aggressive person, they are vexations to the spirit." Of the people that report to hospitals, 80% to 90% come in with stress related illness. Stress was one thing Carol wanted to avoid. When Dean got loud and aggressive, both Carol and Mike disappeared. Then Dean got to "be the store." It worked short term but long term did not work.

156

Carol thought she was preserving her health by keeping her mouth shut and not communicating. "Avoid confrontation at all cost", she thought. This may be correct in some cases but she decided she needed to start speaking up. At first she found herself being screamed at, insulted, degraded with fowl words being hurled at her. It used to be that Dean would be drunk at the store and stumble down the stairs in a drunken stupor. Carol found him lying in his piss and vomit near, the garbage. She found him stumbling down the road many times. Once, she just drove by and let whatever, happen to him, happen. It didn't help to come to his rescue. The police arrived on the scene: another Ticket. By this time Dean discovered that the attorney was just taking his money and doing nothing to influence the courts anyway. He had been spending a lot of money on attorney fees and fines. He crashed a scooter from the store when he was drunk and lost the keys to the store. Carol knew he cared and did his best to make up for the losses that incurred. That does not mean that people should not communicate when they see something needs to change in order to solve the problem.

Once Carol started bringing things to his attention, he came unglued. He felt so bad. He did not want to fight so he asked Mom to go to his therapy session with him to straighten things out.

Dean, Carol and his therapist had a meeting that really lifted his spirits. With Dean's spirits lifted, he became more calm and rejuvenated. If this was the purpose for the outcome of the meeting, it was a big success.

The therapists went with Dean's perceptions. Remember that perceptions are real. They are that person's truth. It doesn't matter what the facts are. It is crucial to work with perceptions to clear any misgivings. We do not have to be right. If the therapist had proceeded with Carols' perceptions or even the facts, it could have never brought about a peaceful outcome.

After Carol became a silent witness and watched what was going on, she had a neutral feeling about things. She did take a look at what went on, didn't say much to Dean afterward but just listened. He began to acknowledge many of the things that Carol had tried to communicate in the past. In the past, before being a silent witness,

157

attempts at communication did not accomplish what they were meant to. After being a silent witness, real communication began.

Whether the therapists had a correct or incorrect picture of what was really happening, it didn't matter. They did know and love the injured soul. They knew how to build on the love, commitment and hard work that Dean was giving. This was what was important. This is what will build this family."

Again, I tell this story to illustrate that we are creating everything we think, say and do. If something doesn't go the way we hope it would, it is still the result of a choice we made, and we should not regret the freedom of our choices.

I also want to express the need to not judge. A head injury and other traumas can cause people to do things that do not make sense; but there is a way. There is always a way. Dean is doing well, and all are learning and growing. All the patience is paying off.

The following story starts out with, but doesn't end with
Positive Thoughts-Positive Actions- Positive Results

Anyone can fall

The family was a deeply religious family. They loved Christ and all his teachings. They were exemplary in every way. Bob was an executive and Dharma a stay at home mom. There were three children: two boys and a girl. Daniel ruled supreme in the house. He cared about everyone and even befriended the underdog. Everyone loved Daniel. He had a wonderful sense of humor, was smart as a whip, and was as handsome as anyone. He was the kind of guy that mothers wanted for their daughters. David was in Daniels' shadow. He never said much and when he did, he stuttered. He was quiet, had a darling smile and fit in, mostly not being noticed much except for the love strokes he got from his mom. He was a gentle child and her love for him was huge. It was a gentle kind love. Angie was the youngest and was treated as the crowning princess in a fairytale. It all seemed real. She was their princess. This was the sort of family everyone wanted to be like. They were the greatest.

158

The family read scriptures together, spent fun time together, worked together and spent play time together. They also had one on one time together. Everything they did appeared perfect. If they were watching a home movie, they stopped the movie if anyone wanted to interject a comment. They listened intently to each person that had something to say and then resumed the movie. Breakfast was made for the children before school and discussions were centered around the days' activities. They took in people that needed a place to stay. Dharma had good things to say to everyone. She would quip, "I'm your good Karma." She thrilled at making people feel good about themselves. She lifted everyone's spirit. Dharma started doing Reiki and energy work. She assisted many people with emotional release. People wanted to 'get rich' so they could give it to Dharma because she did so much for so many people. She was one of the biggest angels I had ever met or had the privilege to know. No one got riches to give to her but she kept on giving. The balance for physical, mental, spiritual was perfection. Their family was whole, complete and perfect. All she did for others will always be remembered with gratitude even with the future events of her life.

It is said that "Pride goeth before the Fall." Did pride, or as Wayne Dyer calls it, "ego," start to set in? I do not know. Dharma said "I've done so many things for so many people. I want something for my self." That, however, in and of itself is harmless. Bob, for the first time after moving, decided to keep the family home from church because he was not asked to be a teacher. He was a "better teacher." Daniel didn't need scouting to learn all those good things. He was already pretty perfect. Almost everyone would agree with him. He would do his good deeds outside of scouting

A friend of Dharmas' had gone though impact training and Dharma could see a big shift in her. She was more confident, self aware and humble. It showed in her posture and countenance. Dharma decided to go. She went through the training with David and a friend. Her friend didn't go to the next level with her group so that she could go to the next level with them.

It was a great experience for all. After they had completed the training, Dharma and her sons wanted to experience all of the trainings they could. Unfortunately, not all trainings are good

Dharma had been leaning toward the new-age way of thinking for a few years. On a trip to Los Angeles, she sought people who were heavy into that thinking. There are many good things about the new-age experience. The music is heavenly, uplifting and calming. Some of the theories were enlightening. No matter what training or religious sect, there are people who take out of it what they want and do not catch the real intent. This family seemed to have adopted the attitude of being against both forms of judgment and that may have contributed to unacceptable behavior. They were totally out of judgment. It may sound good until you take a look at what that might mean. "There is no right or wrong", and everything you do was decided before you got here in life.

Before your soul joined forces with your body, it met with the other little souls. Everyone said what they wanted to do here and the other people said o.k. Example: I want to experience everything life has to offer including rape and murder. Will you let me have my way with you and you say O.K. Then when you get here, you are only doing what you agreed upon before you got here.

What if it went like this? I want to accomplish something that is great and I am going to need your assistance. The experience that I will have, due to who I am going to be born to, may make it difficult for me to accomplish my desire. I am going to this family. It will teach me something because experiences we have will make me stronger but I may or will need support.

Maybe it's like this: I may be a jerk to you because of my DNA and environment so please forgive me and teach me to not be so angry. In return I will be grateful and shower you with love and respect.

I do not believe that anyone plans to do anything hurtful but it might happen because of our weak nature. If you think your soul planned it ahead of time, what would stop you from doing anything hurtful to anyone. It also makes a great cop out.

We are accountable for everything we do. Those who say, "The devil made me do it" or "God told me to" just don't have a grasp on what it is all about. Although I'm not so sure about blame, I am sure about accountability.

160

Daniel told me that he could get into anything: drugs, alcohol, association with criminals and the like and he could come out of it and bring them out with him and thereby save them. Unfortunately, when you associate yourself with a certain element, you can be blamed and even framed.

He once told a friend. "I love you so much that if you went to Hell, I'd go down and get you out."

Daniel may have had good intentions as he started on his road to rescue people. He, being a saint had no idea that he was really on the road to deterioration and the act so vile that it would shatter the lives of many people. Maybe he did know the risk he was taking but wouldn't listen. Maybe it was even subconscious.

A family member had so much trust in this family that when they invited him to come to live with them to rehabilitate him, he said yes and went. Instead of rehabilitating him, the family pulled out the pot and they all stoked.

This family member was on disability and wanted Daniel to be his payee. Daniel saw the free money and decided disability was the way to go. When he didn't have to work anymore and got free money, he wanted more free money. The more money he had the more people he could help.

He started cooking crack in the bathtub. There was great concern. Lives were in danger. It was reported to the police informant line. Even though the police were notified of the activities, they did nothing.

I can not speak from my own experience on the subject of drugs because I have never engaged in any of that scene. I can speak from experience of watching it happen to people I know and people I counseled and people I love.

Drugs alter personalities: they debilitate, they kill and cause one to kill. They make one think irrationally. Beautiful people can fall when influenced by drugs: prescription as well as street drugs.

161

I am saddened by the suffering of families that are affected by senseless acts. I am thankful for those "angels among us" who support and give love and compassion to those who have broken hearts and pray that they will mend. I hope that they can feel the loving arms of God around them to sustain them and give them peace and comfort in what has happened to them.

When my Canyon became an Angel after a tragic accident, I grieved and rejoiced at the same time. I knew where he was and I was thankful for his precious life he had up until that time.

God doesn't make things happen. He allows us to experience and learn. He can only warn us. The warnings are gentle and given with love. He can give us direct warning as well as His warnings found in the scriptures.

Although there is **"No One Thing",** There is "One" thing that can lead us to all good things and that is Jesus Christ. If we will to be like him, we will search the scriptures, be in tune with the Spirit and we will know the truth of all things.

All the things that I have presented in this book, I believe are true. I have made every effort to make no claims. I have given you possibilities of the things that will work for you. It is for you to decide.

Who was it who said he had had no failures? He just found out so many ways that didn't work. He kept trying and found the success.

I have done the same thing with health.

Technology is always changing and I continue to research the latest advances.

SECTION THREE
CHAPTER TWO
WHAT DO YOU CREATE?

There is a popular belief circulating: "No matter what happens to you, you have created it." First of all, if this is true, we have no need to complain, be depressed, blame others or feel sorry for ourselves. If we do not believe it, we can go ahead and do what doesn't work. Complain, be depressed, blame others, feel sorry for ourselves and cause everyone around us to gag and find every excuse to avoid us.

Also if this is true, we can change who we are and be someone we like. A certain young man didn't consciously ask for what happened to him, but subconsciously he may have been willing to go through it. He was ready to shed his ego.

The young man noticed he had acquired a real big ego. He loved to go to the gym, prance around, breathe deeply and prepare to lift his normal weight of over 400 lbs. He recognized that he wanted to be humble but it was a little hard. After all, he was a great trainer, real big and real tough. After thinking about the desire to be humble, but completely forgetting about the interest, a friend happened by and like so many who like to show off their strength, they decided to arm wrestle. They both had really strong muscles: no doubt about it. But this young man didn't know that his bone mass had become less dense. Midway above the elbow on his left arm snapped in half.

He wanted to be humble. He broke his arm. He became humble. But it wasn't that easy. If he hadn't been ready to become humble, he could have turned bitter and angry but he didn't. He could have turned to pain killers and gone through that routine: addiction, unable to function. That was the way it started. He took too much pain medication. He fell and partially paralyzed his right arm. With good support and counseling, he got off all meds, finished his last class to get his bachelors degree, landed a great job and is handling life very well.

With his good thoughts and actions, he created great results

WHAT DO WE REALLY KNOW

A baby girl was born. She was delicate and beautiful. After her Dad went to sleep, her mother sat by the baby's crib for long periods of time while the baby was asleep and tell her how much she loved her. Sometimes it sounded as though the baby was having a hard time breathing. The baby was born early and had weak lungs and so the mother stayed up watching the baby to make sure she stayed breathing and nudged her when she stopped. It was a nightly ritual. There was a nutritional drink that was the only thing that kept the baby from being ill. The mother started getting a little more rest.

The mother was so ill herself and had to fight for her own life a number of times.

The baby girl was growing. Her oldest sibling was extremely cruel to her. The mother did everything she could to keep him away from her.

A number of tragedies happened to individuals in this family. The boys didn't want to be mothered. One thought running the streets was more fun. That affected other siblings. The mother had no control. At least maybe she could save her daughter and youngest son. The three of them took off to beauty pageants and shopping with the money that was awarded the mother to spend in a way that would benefit her daughter because of an accident she was in. The mother let her daughter think that it was the daughters' money. Should have the mother spent the money to draw the family closer? Maybe so. Maybe not. Mother and daughter were very close. The mother never let on that it was a big sacrifice. She chose to love every minute of it.

When her little girl just barely a teen got pregnant there was a family council. She made her decision. She decided to carry the baby full term, have Mom and Dad raise him as their own until she turned 18. Then she would decide if she wanted him to be her son or brother. Mom stopped working, took early childhood classes at the college and opened a day care. Now she could watch the baby so her daughter could stay a kid. No one knew, at that time, with who the baby would eventually be going with, so her parents became the babies Mommy and Daddy.

When the baby was three years old, it looked like the teen was going to keep the baby. Her boyfriend loved him so much There were six months to make the transition from Mommy to Grandma and it happened very smoothly.

The little boy had a new family now. After a while the little boy wanted to be adopted to his dad because the little boy said he wanted to "be connected."

The new little family did not allow mom/grandma be part of the little boy's life. Mom/grandma cried often. It felt like she had not only lost her daughter but also the son/grandson she had raised to that point. It was important for Dad to establish his little family and really bond. It has been done many times that way by many people. The sacrifice was great, but to avoid contention, mom let it rest.

The mom felt tossed aside, accepted it and went on with other important duties. Her sons needed support and unconditional love. She was glad her daughter was being taken care of by a great guy.

The daughter was a great mom. He was a great Dad. The kids were great kids: She had a child with special needs and wanted her mom to be there for her. Mom couldn't go. She was always ill with a cold or flu and was told the baby could die if he was around germs.

Some moms might think, "She dumped me. Why should I bother." or "Oh, my chance to be part of my daughter's life again." or "Oh no, what can I do?" Mom could have thought to go assist but learned out that the child could not be exposed to germs. Mom's flu kept returning, she worked full time, had sons that needed continual support and just felt the challenge had to be her daughters to face.

The daughter had a two-way interaction between her friends and in-laws. There was always support between them. Mom felt the daughter didn't care if she was around but the daughter loved and missed her and suffered the distance between them. Mom learned this only after it may have been too late when it was almost too late.

The bond had been broken between them. Too many years had gone by. A little over 13 years after the mom/grandma lost the little boy, he was killed in a tragic accident.

The grief for mom/grandma was double hard. All the hurt came back from the years of abandonment from her little one and now he, an angel of her life was gone. No one knew her grief.

Her daughter became extremely despondent. She said she couldn't bear it because she lost her son and now she had lost her mother. A counselor told her to forget about her mother, instead of suggesting that she bring her mother in.

It is important for people to make conscious choices and accept the outcome or create a new outcome. It may take time but it is worth it.

Both mother and daughter made choices that brought about the experience; ultimately the bond returned and love is shared again.

Sometimes people need to do things that take their mind off of what ever pain they feel or seek a therapist.

I'm sure you can think of ways that you might have handled it. Maybe you would have started a confrontation and brought it out in the open. It might have caused a better relationship or maybe it would have severed all ties and resulted in a bitter separation.

Sometimes we do for others what we think is best for them because of what is actually best for us.

What ever way you decide to handle something, have no regrets or do something to change it. Repair it if you wish but do not regret it.

You can have anything you want. But remember, you can't have everything you want. It is important to pick and choose the most important things for you. Sometimes you can get a thing that you want but it stops the progress of another thing you want.

If you want to date a certain person passionately, you can.

166

If your higher desire is to be loved, appreciated and respected, you can have that. But if this certain person would bring you misery beyond belief, your higher desire wins out. So never complain.

Your thoughts and your actions will bring certain results.

I worked for the State of Utah. For seven years I had been in a position where I could not use my skills but was so grateful for the paycheck at the end of every 2 weeks that I made sure that I was a team player in my office and did superior work. It was somewhat of a struggle because I was out of character in the office. It was great working there but not without problems. There was no one there I didn't love. Everyone was great. When the office manager position came open I felt a strong feeling that this was my position. I knew that if I didn't get it, I would need to be on my way. When I was overlooked and the new manager came in, I did all I could to make her feel welcome. The other girl in the office, who had been there as long as I, resented the other woman getting hired. She was not very happy that I was supporting the new manager and eventually left the office to find employment elsewhere. The manager told me that the State was trying to get rid of everyone in the office and I was judged by the way the total office ran as a whole. The office was run Laissez-faire because everyone knew their job with their eyes closed. We were not cold, stiff or demanding of others. We just did our jobs and pretty much everyone who came in loved us. For six months I trained the new Office Manager. When my co-worker left, I was o.k. with it because I thought she'd be happier. I was happy for her.

I began to be comfortable in my job and began to rationalize. "I have only 2 ½ years to retirement. "It is a 'piece of cake' here and maybe I'll just stay." I knew that I was supposed to leave (or called elsewhere) but I was too comfortable.

Sometimes, when we disregard what we know and feel to be right and do not act upon it, someone comes into our lives to force the issue. They may be as devious and dishonest as one can imagine. They may get payback another time, but for you, it is what you need at the time.

This new manager who acted like I was wonderful and marvelous for the first approximately eight months, turned like a snake. As soon as we had hired new girl to replace my co-worker in the office, I began being verbally attacked. I was dehumanized, put through character assassination, and my job sabotaged.

I don't know that my character is such that could rant and rave, curse and shout, but I sure understand those who do!

About two weeks after the extreme abuse began, I collapsed at work. The facility nurse summoned. She reported that my blood pressure was 200 over 120. I had two choices: have my husband take me to the emergency room, or she would call the ambulance.

My history has taught me that I am adversely affected by drugs, so I decided to go to a therapist, knowing that mind and body have a distinct correlation.

I found that I, like many people, take on stress by not overtly reacting to negative experience. It manifests itself in physical ways. I learned how to say what I need to say, not holding it to fester, and be honest without the emotion and judgment.

I have learned how to simplify and take care of myself instead of rescuing people unless I know it will not deter mental or physical health.

I did not go back to work. It was time for me to recover.

In my eighth grade yearbook, I recently found, there in print was my desire to be an author or artist. I had completely forgotten about that desire but it makes perfect sense that I researched and saved pertinent information on a number of topics. My life experience has also opened up the way for writing a book to happen. I told God. "If you want me to write a book, it will need to flow." I had written a book a number of years ago and the transcript was lost. That book flowed and I knew I didn't have time to wrestle with another book so I expected God to send his angels to assist me with this one.

168

My goal is to reach people who want to make a difference in their lives and in the lives of their family, friends and neighbors.

The first section of the book was fairly simple. All the therapies that I have learned over the years are second nature to me.

The second section of the book was second nature to me as a child (as with most everyone) but life happened (as with most everyone) and a certain level of doubt, pity and anger set in. I set to work and cleared most of it through therapies.

I have covered some therapies for the mind but I would like to expand on the mind. They are so basic and yet for some, it is extremely difficult because of the mind set they received through DNA and environment. These people who have been shorted good DNA and environment can alter them. "As a man thinketh, so is he" is a scripture and a book by James Allen.

Deepak Chopra says it in a different way in his book 'Creating Affluence' "All of material creation, everything that we can see, touch, hear, taste, or smell is made from the same stuff and comes from the same source. Experiential knowledge of this fact gives us the ability to fulfill any desire we have, acquire any material object we want, and experience fulfillment and happiness to any extent we aspire."......."those same impulses of energy and information that we experience as thought – those same impulses – are the raw material of the universe." Hence, we have the ability to create.

Wayne Dyer says it very well in his book "Intention." Intention is deeper than thought but thought is the first step. The thought comes without effort. You intend to make it happen and proceed with whatever it takes.

The Law of attraction as given in the movie "The Secret" is a great therapy that has not been mentioned in this book. Watch the movie.

I will be listing a number of books at the end of this book. These books have had a significant effect on my life, progress and success. There is great insight in them. They are easily readable and experiences are attainable.

Why are some people able to create Affluence, Love, Health and whatever they want in life and others don't seem to be able to? Mind set.

Children grow up in affluent homes and it is second nature to assume that all will be well with them. Some people grow up in poor homes that they have an insatiable desire to get out of. They "Think and Grow Rich" as Napoleon Hill put it.

If you are down and out, Read, Read, Read: positive books. It will change your mind set. Listen to positive tapes and CD's. Chant or read affirmations. Do energy work.

All you people who are so well adjusted and don't need anything, maybe you *deserve* to be on an even higher plain of existence.

"If ye have the faith of a grain of mustard seed, you can move mountains," say the scriptures. All that we've discussed is simply faith. The way the great authors discuss it, it makes it so logical and simple that exercising faith becomes a reality. If you can get it from the scriptures, there may be no need for this. Or if you apply these things, you may be more likely to understand the scriptures and be able to apply them more fully. It is up to you.

We have the DNA handed down from the beginning. If it is positive DNA, we have strengths. If it is negative DNA we can make it strong by altering it by replacing negative thoughts by practicing strong positive thoughts.

Mind Set

Because of your Heredity/Genes, Environment/Experience, and Spirit, you function in a certain way. All can be changed. There is no reason that you have to stay with what you have and not get what you choose. For some of us, it takes years and total commitment. You can change your DNA by changing your thoughts and actions. Your RNA will go make it happen.

170

RNA

A single-stranded nucleic acid made up of nucleotides. RNA is involved in the transcription of genetic information; the information encoded in DNA is translated into messenger RNA (mRNA), which controls the synthesis of new proteins.

The RNA carries out the command of the DNA.

DNA

Deoxyribonucleic acid. DNA molecules carry the genetic information necessary for the organization and functioning of most living cells and control the inheritance of characteristics.

The DNA stores the information of the entire human structure including thoughts. Layers of Light Products can erase the effects of negative thought.

Thus, even the thoughts we think are in our DNA and if the RNA is working properly, it gets the job done.

So all you scientific enthusiasts can now know that your thoughts create the outcome.

How do we end up with our thoughts?

Again, we get our thoughts by way of the three things stated above: Heredity, Environment and Spirit.

How can we change our thoughts?

Reading, Therapies, and Service (the best form of experience).

Years ago, I assumed that my husband could do something or other. He got really irritated with me. I couldn't figure out why he got so upset. In his mind, was I mocking his inability to do it? Was he being stubborn because he didn't want to do it for me? Maybe I wasn't worth it. Or maybe he just didn't think he could do it and I was pestering him to do something he knew he could not do.

171

My faith in him resulted in unpleasantness but I continued to have faith in him and he started doing things he didn't even think he could do and he was so impressed with his projects. That is great.

There is a saying that goes something like this:

The past is history; the future is a mystery; the present is a gift from God. That is why we call it the present.

There are other versions but I prefer this one

If you are living in or dwelling on the past, you are simply not taking advantage of what the present offers. Your conversation gives you away. You continually speak fondly or bitterly about the things that you loved or loathed. You may even drum up excuses for why you are the way you are. You are letting the present opportunities escape you.

To live in the past is not productive or satisfying. To dwell on it causes you to miss out on life: literally. It causes you to miss out on the opportunities of today.

If something from the past pops up to give you a smile or causes a grateful reminder, it is harmless.

If you have issues relating to past experiences, there is a time and place for clearing them. Seek assistance from a professional. See my section on therapies.

The future is a mystery, so why concern yourself with it? Do what you can today and do the best you can. The future will take care of itself.

Most people do not know ahead of time what may happen tomorrow to change everything in their lives. When that happens and it is today, you handle it. You make choices.

Births, deaths. marriages, employment and tragedy are all things that cause a sudden change. Planning for the future is important:

172

college, job choices and friendships etc are important, however, be flexible and open to change at any time.

The present is truly a gift from God. In a sense, it is all there is. Today you can choose.

The truth of what I am saying is found in Bruce Lipton's DVD "The New Biology: Where Mind and Body Meet." It is available through Spirit 2000, Inc. 1 800 550-5571 or visit www.brucelipton.com or www.spirit2000.com   Address Sprit 2000, Inc. P.O. Box 41126 Memphis, TN 38174-1126

"Recent advances in cellular science are heralding an important evolution turning point. For almost fifty years we have held the illusion that our health and fate were preprogrammed in our genes, a concept referred to as Genetic Determinacy.   Though mass consciousness is currently imbued with the belief that the character of one's life is genetically predetermined, a radical new understanding is unfolding at the leading edge of science. Cellular biologists now recognize that the environment – the external universe and our internal physiology – and more importantly, our perception of the environment, directly control the activity of our genes.

An awareness of how vibrational signatures and resonance impact molecular communication constitutes a master key that unlocks a mechanism by which our thoughts, attitudes and beliefs create the conditions of our body and the external world.

The truth is that genes are selected and rewritten by our belief systems.

Before the 1600's the mission statement of science was: "To gain an understanding of the natural order so that we can live in harmony with it."

But in the 1600's the modern science mission statement became "To obtain knowledge that can be used to dominate and control nature." This is just the tip off the iceberg. See his research by checking out his web site given above.

HONESTY

In "touch for health," a muscle is pressed after a statement is said. If the muscle goes weak, the statement is not true (the answer is NO). If the muscle is strong, the answer is true (the answer is YES). There are things that cause it to not work properly such as being dehydrated or goofing around with it but that is not the point I am making at this time. Bottom line is. When you lie, your muscles go weak even if your conscious self does not know it is a lie.

What is a muscle? All the organs in your body are muscles. If your muscles weaken, is that a contribution to ill-health? I believe it does.

I know that there are times when you would rather have your muscles weaken than to have someone rant and rave, insult and degrade. This can be an even greater energy drain. Avoid these people or spend less time with them if you can. The more you can stay away from energy draining people and not let them into your thoughts and actions, the better health you can have. Some people have little ability to express anything that seems to be of value and is completely boring or worse: irritating. This can also be energy draining, stressful and unhealthy. Make choices but do not judge

There is another kind of person that speaks well, uplifts and just makes you feel incredible. You can enjoy listening to a good orator but you do not have to buy into what they are saying. The Power of the Word is good and it is capable of impressing the world. It says nothing about the person behind the words. We have some people who have that gift to open their mouth and everything that comes out seems like gold. Admire them for their talent but do not assume that everything they say is true. Make choices but do not judge.

I have had the pleasure of knowing both types of people. I enjoy listening to a speaker. I do not enjoy listening to a boring conversation but I can and do enjoy other obvious qualities of that person. I can listen to the person without listening to the words and when something is said that I can respond do, I can hear that.

Everyone has gifts to give and gifts to receive. One can not happen without the other. A gift does not even have to be tangible: love, gratitude, a smile and acknowledgement are some that require nothing but an attitude.

YOU ARE RIGHT

There is a saying. "If you think it is, you are right. If you think it isn't, you are right." Your thoughts are actually creating the result, so if you want something good to happen, believe it. You are right.

Someone else said if you think that life should be perfect, you will be disappointed. If you do not expect everything to be perfect, you won't be disappointed when life happens.

If you think that life sucks and life isn't fair, you are right. So get over the pity party and just deal with it (unless you are enjoying the misery).

I'm sure you can think of a lot of reasons you can pity yourself. Get off that thought and think of all the things that you are thankful for. If you can't think of anything, be ware. You may lose something you took for granted. Even people who have lost body parts or who are mentally challenged have great accomplishments.

I use to weep over people that had a lot of excess fat on their bodies. I've changed my mind. They have it for a reason. Some have been molested and can not handle looking good. It is a real threat. Some husbands are terrified that they will loose their wife if she looks too good so he creates it. He brings her candies. Some people think food is love. If they do not get the love they need, they eat. Most of the reasons are deep seeded issues that they are not aware of.

There are therapies for issues. They are covered in Section I. Some refer to these therapies as inner work. As I said at the beginning of this section, mental has a profound influence on physical. I may or may not have covered this adequately but this work creates miracles. I have used a number of healers doing energy work and I have seen so much. It grieves me that there are not more people taking advantage of these healing modalities. It is important that you feel

175

comfortable with these service providers before you even make any commitments other than a free consultation. Phone can be adequate communication and for some therapies. Ask for fees. Some will do part trade but the first rule is to feel comfortable with the person. Trust. Sometimes you may not feel a shift at first. If you pay close attention during the coming week you may notice a subtle change and sometimes a major shift happens.

.

STORIES OF HIGHER AWARENESS

I pass along to you by open permission, on an e-mail exchange on the internet. Bill Graham's daughter, Anne Graham Lotz, was interviewed on the Early Show and Jane Clayson asked her "How could God let something like this happen?" regarding the attacks of Sept ll. She gave an extremely Profound and insightful response:

She said, "I believe God is deeply saddened by this, just as we are, but for years we've been telling God to get out of our schools, to get out of our government and to get out of our lives. And being the gentleman He is, I believe He has calmly backed out. How can we expect God to give us His blessing and His protection if we demand He leave us alone?" In light of recent events...terrorists attacks, school shootings, etc. I think it started when atheist Madeleine Murray O'Hare (She was murdered, her body found recently) complained she didn't want prayer in our schools. And we said OK.

Then someone said you better not read the Bible in school... the Bible says thou shalt not kill, thou shalt not steal, and love your neighbor as yourself. And we said OK. The Dr. Benjamin Spock said we shouldn't spank our children when they misbehave because their little personalities would be warped and we might damage their self-esteem (Dr. Spock's son committed suicide). We said an expert should know what he's talking about. And we said OK.

Then someone said teachers and principals better not discipline our children when they misbehave. The school administrators said no faculty member in this school better touch a student when they misbehave because we don't want any bad publicity, and we surely don't want to be sued (there's a big difference between disciplining, touching, beating, smacking, humiliating, kicking, etc. and we said OK.

Then someone said, let's let our daughters have abortions if they want, and they won't even have to tell their parents. And we said OK.

Then some wise school board member said, since boys will be boys and they're going to do it anyway, let's give our sons all the condoms they want so they can have all the fun they desire, and we won't have to tell their parents they got them at school. And we said OK.

Then some of our top elected officials said it doesn't matter what we do in private as long as we do our jobs. Agreeing with them, we said it doesn't matter to me what anyone, including the President, does in private as long as I have a job and the economy is good. Then someone said let's print magazines with pictures of nude women and call it wholesome, down-to-earth appreciation of the beauty of the female body. And we said OK.

And then someone else took that appreciation a step further and published pictures of nude children and then further again by making them available on the internet. And we said OK; they're entitled to free speech. Then the entertainment industry said; let's make TV shows and movies that promote profanity, violence, and illicit sex. Let's record music that encourages rape, drugs, murder, suicide, and satanic themes. And we said it's just entertainment, it has no adverse effect, nobody takes it seriously anyway. So go right ahead. Now we're asking ourselves why our children have no conscience, why they don't know right from wrong, and why it doesn't bother them to kill strangers, their classmates, and themselves. Probably, if we think about it long and hard enough, we can figure it out. I think it has a great deal to do with "WE REAP WHAT WE SOW."

Unfortunately, is seems so simple for people to trash God and then wonder why the world's going to hell. Why do we believe what the newspapers say, but question what The Bible says? How many people send 'jokes' through e-mail which spread like wildfire, but are afraid to send messages regarding the Lord because they are afraid of what people might think? It is sad how lewd, crude, vulgar and obscene articles pass freely through cyberspace, but public discussion of God is suppressed in the school and workplace.

How can we be more worried about what other people think of us, than what God thinks of us."

It is good to see people speak up for truth with wisdom and courage. Anne Graham Lotz, did a superb job. As she wished, I am passing it along.

There is a way to stand up for truth and goodness. We can condemn the act but not the person. We can give unconditional love to those who make others lives miserable.

If you can not deal with it don't be around it. If you want and are able to make a difference in someone's life and change the outcome of the future that is commendable.

There are two stories about doing something different and creating a positive outcome. One is entitled: "Who I Am Makes a Difference." The other is entitled, "One Small Action."

Who I Am Makes A Difference

A teacher decided to honor each of her seniors in high school telling them the difference they each made. She called each student to the front of the class, one at a time. First she told each of them how they had made a difference to her and the class. Then she presented each of them with a blue ribbon imprinted with gold letters, which read, "Who I am makes a difference."

Afterwards the teacher decided to do a class project to see what kind of impact recognition would have on a community. She gave each of the students three more ribbons and instructed them to go out and spread this acknowledgment ceremony. Then they were to follow up on the results, see who honored whom and report back to the class in about a week.

One of the boys in the class went to a junior executive in a nearby company and honored him for helping him with his career planning. He gave him a blue ribbon and put it on his shirt. Then he handed him two extra ribbons and said, "We're doing a class project on recognition. We'd like you to go out and find somebody to honor, give them a blue ribbon, then give them the extra blue ribbon so they can acknowledge a third person to keep this acknowledgement ceremony going. Then please report back to me and tell me what happened."

Later that day the junior executive went in to see his boss, who had been noted, by the way, as being kind of a grouchy fellow. He sat his boss down and he told him that he deeply admired him for being a creative genius. The boss seemed very surprised. The junior executive asked him if he would accept the gift of the blue ribbon and would he give him permission to put it on him. His surprised boss said, "Well, sure." The junior executive took the blue ribbon and placed it right on the boss's jacket above his heart. As he gave him the last extra ribbon, he said, "Would you do me a favor? Would you take this extra ribbon and pass it on by honoring somebody else? The young boy who first gave me the ribbons is doing a project in school and we want to keep this recognition ceremony going and find out how it affects people."

That night the boss came home to his 14-year-old son and sat him down. He said, "The most incredible thing happened to me today. I was in my office and one of the junior executives came in and told me he admired me and gave me a blue ribbon for being a creative genius. Imagine. He thinks I'm a creative genius. Then he put this blue ribbon that says 'Who I Am Makes a Difference', on my jacket above my heart. He gave me an extra ribbon and asked me to find somebody else to honor. As I was driving home tonight, I started thinking about whom I would honor with this ribbon and I thought about you. I want to honor you. My days are really hectic and when I come home I don't pay a lot of attention to you. Sometimes I scream at you for not getting enough good grades in school and for your bedroom being a mess, but somehow tonight, I just wanted to sit here and, well, just let you know that you do make a difference to me. Besides your mother, you are the most important person in my life. You're a great kid and I love you!"

The startled boy started to sob and sob, and he couldn't stop crying. His whole body shook. He looked up at his father and said through his tears, "Dad, earlier tonight I sat in my room and wrote a letter to you and mom explaining why I had killed myself and asking you to forgive me. I was going to commit suicide tonight after you were asleep. I just didn't think that you cared at all. The letter is upstairs.
180

I don't think I need it after all." His father walked upstairs and found a heart felt letter full of anguish and pain. The envelope was addressed, "Mom and Dad."

The boss went back to work a changed man. He was no longer a grouch but made sure to let all his employees know that they made a difference. The junior executive helped several other young people with career planning and never forgot to let them know that they made a difference in his life...one being the boss's son. And, the young boy and his classmates learned a valuable lesson. Who you are DOES make a difference?

ONE SMALL ACTION

One day, when I was a freshman in high school, I saw a kid from my class walking home from school His name was Kyle. It looked as if he were carrying all of his books.

I thought to myself, "Why would anyone bring home all his books on a Friday?" "He must really be a nerd."

I had quite a weekend planned (parties and a football game with friends), so I shrugged my shoulders and went on, but then I saw a bunch of kids running toward him. They tripped him, and as he fell into the dirt, all the books flew out of his arms. His glasses went flying, and I saw them land in the grass about ten feet from him. As he looked up, I saw this terrible sadness in his eyes.

My heart went out to him, so I jogged over. I could see tears in his eyes as he crawled around looking for his glasses. "Those guys are jerks," I said, as I handed him his glasses. "They need to get-a-life!"

He looked at me and said, "Hey, thanks!" There was a big smile on his face. It was one of those smiles that showed real gratitude.

As we gathered his books, I asked him where he lived. It turned out, he lived near me. I asked him why I'd never seen him before. He informed me he'd been going to a private school. In my mind, a kid from a private school would not be my choice to hang out with. I carried some of his books, and we talked all the way to his home. He turned out to be a pretty cool kid.

I asked him if he wanted to play a little football with me and my friends. Of course, his answer was yes, and we hung out all weekend. The more my friends and I got to know Kyle, the more we liked him.

Monday morning came, and there was Kyle lugging the huge stack of books back to school. I stopped him and said, "Boy, you are gonna really build some serious muscles with this pile of books!" He just laughed and handed me half the books. Over the next four years, Kyle and I became best friends.

At last we were seniors. Upon graduation, Kyle would be going to Georgetown University, and planned to become a doctor. I teased him about being a big nerd. I was going to Duke University on a football scholarship and major in business. No matter how many miles separated us, I knew we would always be friends.

It was graduation day. I caught a glimpse of Kyle. He looked great. He had really found himself during high school. He had filled out, and actually looked good in glasses. He had more dates than I had, and all the girls loved him. Boy, sometimes I was jealous! Today was one of those days.

Kyle was valedictorian of our class, so he would be speaking. He was nervous. I smacked him on the back and said, "Hey, big guy, you'll do great!" He looked at me with one of those looks (the really grateful one) and smiled. "Thanks," he said. When it was time for his speech, I watched, as he strode confidently to the podium. He cleared his throat emotionally, and paused for a moment looking down. He then raised his head scanning the audience, and began.

"Graduation is a time to thank those who helped you make it through these tough years, your parents, your teachers, your siblings, maybe a coach…but mostly your friends…and his eye rested for a moment on me. I am here to tell all of you, that being a friend to someone is the very best gift you can give. Here is my story.

As I listened, my thoughts turned to shock and disbelief. I heard the gasps go through the crowd, as this handsome, popular boy told us about his weakest moment. He began relating, in detail, the event that had transpired on the first day we met.

He had planned to kill himself over that weekend. He spoke of how he had cleaned out his locker so his Mom wouldn't have to do it later, and was carrying his stuff home. He looked directly at me, and gave me a little smile. Thankfully, a kid, and his one small act of kindness, saved me from doing the unspeakable. He has become my best friend.

His mom and dad were looking at me, smiling with gratitude. Not until that moment did I realize the depth of my actions. With one seemingly small gesture, you can change a person's life.

Report on Quantum Physics

This report is given to bring awareness to possibilities, new to some, though there is much available on this subject. This is only a fraction but it is important to realize that Science and Technology is out there working for you and me. **Layers of Light** puts the science of classical and quantum discoveries together and creates a most remarkable tool for Health and Wellness. The movie: **"The Secret"** goes into Quantum Physics beautifully. I hope you enjoy.

The Following compilation was organized by R. Neil Voss. It is pretty Awesome. This will put your mind to thinking.

THE ELECTROMAGNETIC SPECTRUM:

Most of what we refer to as "energy" is all or some part of the electromagnetic spectrum. The electromagnetic spectrum consists of various types or forms of energy including heat, light, infrared light, ultraviolet light, radio and television waves, microwaves, x-rays, and gamma rays. More specifically, the electromagnetic spectrum is made up of energy waves that travel and spread out or "radiate" as they travel.

The energies of the electromagnetic spectrum consist of moving waves of varying frequencies. The higher the frequency, the faster the wave of energy is moving. And faster waves move more quickly because they "possess" more energy. The faster the wave, the more energy it contains.

In addition to frequency (measured as cycles per second or Hertz), the energies of electromagnetic spectrum can be measured as wavelengths (meters) and as energy (electron volts).

When speaking of the electromagnetic spectrum, we usually refer to its energies as waves with varying frequencies. However, the energies of the spectrum can also be conceptualized as matter-like particles or subatomic particles. In the physical universe, waves and particles have distinctly different characteristics or behaviors.

For example, waves of visible light may be said to consist of particles called "photons." Sometimes visible light appears as if it were made of photons and displays the characteristics of particles or matter. At other times visible light displays the characteristics expected of waves.

The waves or vibrations of the electromagnetic spectrum penetrate both space and matter. Matter consists of atoms, and atoms consist of subatomic particles of energy. These subatomic particles, such as protons, electrons, and neutrons are in constant motion, and therefore, the atoms they create are in constant motion too. If the motion of the atoms and its subatomic particles were to stop or cease, the subatomic particles would "fall" into or be drawn into

184

each other, destroying the atoms as well as the matter created by the atoms.

When electromagnetic waves penetrate matter, they can add to or increase the energy of the subatomic particles thus increasing the motion of the subatomic particles and the motion of the atoms that make up the matter of an object. For example, when a heated object is applied to some part of the body, the heat radiates into that body part, increasing the energy of atoms of the particular body part. The end result is that the body part feels warmer

However, if the electromagnetic waves deliver too much energy to the body part, the motion of the subatomic particles increases and the particles escape the atoms, causing the atoms to disintegrate or combine with other types of atoms. The end result is that the body part is burned or destroyed.

In addition to electromagnetic waves, we are surrounded by waves or vibrations carried by matter. Explosions, earthquakes, and animal stampedes cause solid matter to vibrate. Tossing a stone into a lake creates waves in water. Waves carried by the air (a combination of gasses) produce sounds, including human speech

As human animals, we have specialized sensory organs that detect certain ranges or frequencies of waves. Our eyes detect what we call visible light. Our ears pick up waves in the air. We have a variety of receptors that detect waves and momentum in solid objects like the Earth and escalators.

There are many wave frequencies for which our bodies lack receptors, such as radio waves, microwaves, ultraviolet light, x-rays, and gamma rays to name a few. Just because we cannot sense such frequencies does not mean that these rays do not affect us. Over-exposure to such rays can result in burns, sickness, and death.

As mentioned earlier, we are surrounded and penetrated by a multitude of waves. Waves are everywhere, and they crisscross or collide with one another constantly. Waves of similar frequencies may combine, producing waves of new frequencies. Whatever the end result, when waves produced by two or more sources cross one

185

another, they may interfere with one another. The resulting new patterns are referred to as "interference patterns."

HOLOGRAPHY AND HOLOGRAPHS:

The English word " holography" literally means "complete writing," and is derived from a combination of the early Greek words "holo" (whole) and "graph" (written).

"Holography" is used to refer to the idea that every part of a "writing" or written form or graphic image contains information about the whole or entire document, written production, or image.

A "holograph" or "hologram" is the physical form or manifestation of holography.

"Holographs" are three-dimensional photographs made with laser beams. To make the original holograph, the beam of a laser is split into two beams by a partially reflective mirror. One of the two split beams is then projected onto the object to be photographed. The object reflects the beam onto the photographic plate or film. The other part of the split beam is reflected directly onto the same photographic plate.

When the two parts of the original laser beam strike the photographic plate, a picture of seemingly meaningless, curvy lines appears on the plate. This pattern of lines is referred to as an "interference pattern." Whenever the "interference pattern" on the plate is illumined by a laser beam, a three-dimensional image of the original photographed object appears.

PROPERTIES OF HOLOGRAPHS:

Holographs have many properties or behaviors that are absent in normal photographs. For example, a normal photograph produces a two-dimensional image, in which depth is merely inferred; the image produced by a holograph is three-dimensional and may appear to be as real as the original object.

186

With a normal photograph, there is a one-to-one correspondence between the points on the photograph and the image it contains. For example, in a photograph of a human being, the image of the head is recorded in one specific place or part of the photograph, and the image of the torso is recorded in a specific part of the photograph that corresponds to where we would expected it to be. The same is true for the arms, legs, etc. The part of the photograph that contains the head will always contain the head. The same is true for the rest of the body and photograph. The head always contains the head and nothing else. If the part of the photograph containing the head is cut off, the head is gone.

Holographs contain the entire photographed image throughout the entire holograph. If the holograph is cut into two pieces, each piece contains the entire image. Cutting it into three pieces produces three complete images. Four pieces produce four holographs, etc. The entire image is contained throughout the holograph in the wavy lines of the interference pattern. Due to the current state of holography, as the holograph is cut into more and more smaller and smaller pieces, the image begins to lose detail and clarity. It is believed that this loss is due to the materials used for holographs. Ideally, a holograph can be cut infinitely and still contain the entire image of the object.

This characteristic of holographs, their unusual relationship between the whole and its parts, suggests that information contained within the whole of a holograph is simultaneously shared with its parts. Albert Einstein's theory of relativity limits the exchange of energy, matter, or information to the speed of light. The more recent theory of quantum physics predicts that the exchange of energy, matter, and information throughout the universe is instantaneous, not limited by the speed of light. Recent technological developments in the field of physics support the instantaneous exchange of information, which is consistent with a holographic model of the universe.

Another very interesting property of holographs is that an extremely large number of different images can be recorded on the same photographic plate without interfering with one another. Holographs can record and store an astounding number of separate holographic images if the angles of the reflected laser beams striking the film are changed. It is possible to record many different images on the same surface by slight changes in the angles of the beams. It has been demonstrated that one cubic centimeter of film can hold as many as 10 billion bits of information. The image that appears when the holograph is illuminated depends on which interference pattern is illumined. The choice of interference patterns is determined by characteristics of the illuminating laser beam such as its angle, depth, or frequency. The ability to store an almost infinite number of images or information in much the same space serves as a model for the storage of information in the human brain.

Holographs also allow images to mix or blend under certain circumstances, which also serves as a model for the human brain's creativity and other similar processes and as a model for psychedelic and psychotherapeutic experiences.

HOLISM AND THE HOLONOMIC APPROACH:

The group of principles referred to as "holonomic," "holographic," "hologram," or "hologrammic" refer to an alternative approach to the conventional understanding of the relationship between the whole and its parts, transcending the conventional distinctions between the whole and its parts.

The scientist/philosopher Smuts best stated the characteristics of the holonomic approach in his philosophy of "Holism":

1) Holism regards all organic things as wholes, not just assemblages of parts;
2) The whole and its parts mutually and reciprocally influence and change each other;
3) Every whole possesses its inner order or pattern, as well as being a part of a more extensive pattern.

HOLOGRAPHIC MODEL OF MEMORY AND THE BRAIN AS A HOLOGRAM:

For thousands of years, philosophers, educators, scientists, biologists, neurologists, neuro-psychologists, psychologists, and brain specialists have speculated about memory and how the human

188

brain stores and retrieves information. As advances in anatomy and physiology were being made in the late 1800's, several theories were proposed to account for the function of memory. One theory held that each memory or unit of memory was encoded in a single neuron in the brain. Another theory speculated that memories were stored by a group of neurons working together. Still another theory proposed that memories were stored in units called "engrams." Most theories proposed that every memory was stored in a specific location and that if the location was damaged, the memory would be lost forever.

The theories of specific locations, or localized memory, are supported to a great extent by observations of internal and external brain damage and disease. Brain damage caused by striking the head in specific regions with heavy and/or sharp objects tend to cause similar memory losses in most individuals. Strokes, aneurisms, and brain tumors do likewise. However, if the victim lives, another part of the brain may eventually retrieve what was lost.

For decades numerous studies have shown that memories are dispersed throughout the brain instead of being confined to one particular location. In the 1920s, brain scientist Karl Lashley searched for the location of engrams and for the specific locations of memories of learned, complex tasks in rats. He found that no matter what part of the brain he removed and that no matter how much of the brain he removed, the rats could still perform the complex tasks. The memories of how to perform the specific tasks seemed to be throughout the brain and that the memories were not dependent on any particular amount of brain matter. That is, the memories were present throughout the brain and were completely intact in even the minute amounts of brain matter. The whole memory was stored in every part no matter how small the part. None of the available models of memory storage and brain function were able to account for Lashley's findings.

Currently, it is believed that the average human brain consists of millions of neurons and is capable of storing at least 10 billion bits of information. The quantity of stored information far exceeds the number of neurons as well as their possible connections and groupings.

In the 1960's neuro-psychologist Karl Pribram applied the holographic model to the process of memory storage in the human brain. He found that the processes of storing, retrieving, and combining information were similar to the techniques of optical holography. Pribram proposed that memories are encoded in the brain by means of patterns of nerve impulses that crisscross the entire brain in the same way that interference patterns crisscross an entire piece of holographic encoded film.

Pribram further proposed that the brain itself is a hologram which can contain extraordinary amounts of information within very little space. In a hologram the same image or information is found throughout the hologram, and every image or bit of information stored in the hologram is interconnected with all other images and bits of information. Therefore, it is not necessary to go through all images and bits of information in a particular order to retrieve a memory. All memories are connected and can be used to retrieve a specific memory when needed. When the human brain is retrieving a particular memory, it does not follow any logical, linear sequence of categories. The interconnectedness of all stored information allows for almost instantaneous recall. Following Pribram's lead, other experimental psychologists applied the holographic model to the processes of perception and movement and were able to account for phenomena that could not be explained by the current psycho-physiological theories.

QUANTUM THEORY:

By the end of the 1920's, physicists had developed a largely theoretical body of thought known as quantum mechanics or quantum theory to explain a number of observed oddities in the behavior of subatomic particles (Neumann, 1931). Quantum theory postulated that reality consisted of only observed phenomena, that reality did not exist separately from or independently of observation, that quantum mechanics could explain all of the peculiarities of subatomic particles, and that there was no deeper reality underlying quantum theory.

190

ALAIN ASPECT AND NONLOCALITY:

In 1982 French physicist Alain Aspect and his associates at the University of Paris were able to prove through experimentation that under certain circumstances subatomic particles such as electrons are able to communicate instantaneously with one another regardless of the distance separating them (Talbot, 1991). Electrons reacted instantaneously to each other even if they were billions of miles apart. Each seemed to know what the other was doing.

Before Aspect's experiment, physicists believed Albert Einstein's assumption that communication between any two particles in the universe could not occur faster than the speed of light. For physicists, the instantaneous communication between subatomic particles meant that their understanding of and beliefs about the nature of the universe were inaccurate at some level.

The results of Aspect's experiment meant that subatomic particles were connected to one another non-locality. That is, at the level of subatomic particles, space or distance did not exist. Earlier physicists had believed that no two objects could occupy the same space at the same time. This new concept of non-locality meant that everything was happening in the same place at the same time.

Although non-locality was a new concept for most Western scientists, it is an ancient one that serves as an experiential foundation for most mystical experiences, for many aboriginal religions, for the religions of the south central Asian Vedic traditions, for Taoism in China, for idealist philosophies like those of Plato, for para-psychological phenomena, for much occult philosophy, metaphysical teachings, and for most "New Thought" and "New Age" religions. Richard Bach expresses the concept of non-locality in his many writings, and it is the main theme of his "No Such Place As Far Away" (1979). Non-locality is a major theme of the many books that Jane Roberts' books channeled from "Seth.." Non-locality is explained most humorously In her book, The Education of Oversoul Seven (1973).

THE QUANTUM POTENTIAL:

Physicist David Bohm (1980) was particularly drawn to quantum theory, but he arrived at different conclusions about reality at the quantum level. He hypothesized that at the quantum level there existed wave-like phenomena manifesting between electrons in what had previously been thought of as empty space. He believed that these waves, unlike electromagnetic waves, were independent of the laws of physical time and space. He referred to this wave-like information field as the quantum potential and postulated that the quantum potential provided electrons with information about the environment.

Bohm believed that, while the quantum potential possessed possibly an infinite amount of energy, it was not the energetic characteristics of the quantum potential that changed the course of the electrons or caused them to behave in any particular way. Instead, the quantum potential provided guidance or information for electrons. Because the quantum potential depended only on its form or informational-providing characteristics and not on its intensity, its effect on electrons and other subatomic particles did not diminish over space or time. The quantum potential communicated information instantaneously to all particles everywhere and was not limited by the speed of light, the upper limit for the speed of signals proposed by Albert Einstein. The quantum potential could be seen as providing information from a meta-physical realm beyond the confines of space and time.

THE BASIS OF REALITY -- CONSCIOUSNESS:

Bohm proposed that consciousness was the ultimate basis of reality, that matter and energy were created by consciousness, and that all matter and energy contain some degree of consciousness. The qualities of consciousness exist in all matter, right down to subatomic particles. Bohm proposed that electrons possessed a degree of intelligence of their own.

Bohm hypothesized that electrons and all subatomic particles have some degree of consciousness, that every part of reality at every level has its own degree of consciousness, and that the smallest
192

building blocks of the universe are not matter, atoms, subatomic particles, or energy, but instead consciousness. He concluded that consciousness is the basis of reality, that matter and energy are created by consciousness, that consciousness creates reality, and that consciousness creates its own experience of the reality that it creates.

Bohm believed that the consciousness of electrons freely use the information from the quantum potential to choose one particular outcome out of a possible infinity of outcomes. Thus, in one laboratory the electrons might choose an outcome that is completely different from the choices of electrons in other laboratories.

ORDER VERSUS CHANCE, RANDOMNESS AND UNCERTAINTY:

Because electrons have choices and because they choose certain outcomes in some situations and different outcomes in other situations, their behavior was considered to be due to "chance," "randomness," and "uncertainty." Bohm postulated that such "chance" outcomes were actually determined by a realm of variables which underlie quantum reality. He proposed that this "deeper" level of reality was purposefully choosing the outcomes and that what appeared as chance or randomness was meaningful and purposeful when understood in terms of the underlying reality. Bohm referred to the observable (observable by the physical senses or by technical extensions of these senses) universe as the "explicate order" and the underlying, unobservable reality that produced the observable universe as the "implicate order."

THE EXPLICATE ORDER AND THE IMPLICATE ORDER:

Dr. Bohm believed that Aspect's experiment proved that objective reality does not exist. He also believed that Aspect's results provided evidence the universe was really a gigantic hologram consisting of two orders of reality: an "explicate order" and an "implicate order," as mentioned above. The explicate order, also referred to as the unfolded order, consists of the physical or manifested reality which can be detected by our physical senses or by the technological extensions of our senses. The implicate order, or enfolded order, consists of a deeper, more vast, underlying order out of which the explicate order arises.

All of the phenomena of our physical universe are made up of atoms. Atoms consist of smaller or subatomic particles such as electrons, protons, and neutrons. Technical advances in physics have allowed us to observe subatomic particles to some degree. We find that subatomic particles are in constant motion, that they seem to vanish and that "newly" created particles appear.

According to Bohm, subatomic particles dissolve into the implicate order and new particles arise from the implicate order. However, physicists falsely perceive subatomic particles as separate entities. According to Bohm, all subatomic particles are merely ripples in the continuous structure of the implicate order. The vanished subatomic particles are not lost because they are just as much a part of the implicate order as they were when we mistakenly perceived them as independent. The newly created subatomic particles, which appear to be separate entities, are really ripples in the implicate order and have never separated from it. The subatomic particles such as electrons and protons are ripples in the fabric of the implicate order.

THE HOLOGRAPHIC UNIVERSE:

Bohm hypothesized that subatomic particles appear to be separate objects because we are seeing only a portion of reality. He proposed that subatomic particles are part of a deeper, underlying unity that is indivisible and holographic. Since the apparent separateness of subatomic particles is illusory and everything in physical reality is composed of subatomic particles, the apparent separateness of things in the physical universe is illusory, everything is interconnected, and the physical universe is a holographic projection of the deeper, underlying reality. The Bhagavad-Gita (7:6-7) describes a similar model of reality, "The birth and dissolution of the cosmos itself take place in me. There is nothing that exists separate from me, Arjuna. The entire universe is suspended from me as my necklace of jewels."

Bohm believed that all subatomic particles throughout the universe are connected to one another because they are all interconnected
194

parts or projections of the implicate order. Thus, at the subatomic or quantum level, all particles are part of the implicate order, interconnected, and constantly communicating with one another. Since the explicate order is a holographic projection the implicate order, all physical or manifested objects are connected and in communication with all parts of the explicate order even though they appear to be separate objects.

Bohm proposed that every part of this holographic universe contains all the information possessed by the whole. If the universe is a holograph, then every particle of the universe contains information concerning the entire universe. The whole is present in every part. In fact, there are no "parts." The perception of parts or separate objects or categories is an illusion which is created by the human mind and by human language, but which helps us operate within the explicate order.

Again from the Vedic/Hindu tradition, we find in the Shvetashvatara Upanishad, a poetic description of the wholeness of the universe, connected through an underlying reality, "May the Lord of Love, who projects himself into this universe of myriad forms, from whom all beings come and to whom all return, grant us the grace of wisdom. He is fire and the sun, and the moon and the stars. He is the air and the sea, and the Creator, Prajapati. He is this boy, he is that girl, he is this man, he is that woman, and he is this old man, too, tottering on his staff. His face is everywhere."

REALITY AS PROCESSES AND HOLOMOVEMENT:

The human brain and most human languages describe the universe as one full of objects or things. However, all manifested "material" things are actually processes in constant motion not only at the atomic and subatomic levels, but at all levels. Reality consists of constantly changing processes. Some seem to change slower than others, and the human mind has found it helpful to describe many processes, such as mountains, trees, grass, animals, and other humans as solid, static things instead of as ever-changing processes which comprise the ever-changing explicate and implicate realities. Since the term "hologram" generally refers to a static image, Bohm

195

preferred to describe the universe as a "holomovement" in order to capture the continually active and changing nature of reality.

At the quantum level, the universe is not just changing, though. It is continually and constantly disappearing and reappearing. The universe, or the subatomic particles that make up the universe, is/are continually arising from the implicate order and dissolving back into it. The sparks of energy/matter that make up our physical being and our world are continuously appearing and disappearing and being "replaced," so to speak, by newly formed particles.

THE ETERNAL NOW:

Time is just as holographic as space. Within the holographic universe the past, present, and the future all exist simultaneously. Not only does everything interpenetrate everything else spatially, but temporally as well. The concepts of time and space are meaningless to a holographic or holomoving universe, and this is especially true at the deeper implicate level.

According to Bohm, each part contains the information not only of "space," but of "time" as well. That is, the past, present, and future of all parts of the holographic universe can be found in each part. The past, present, and future are happening in this same "space" or "location" and all of time can be found in each moment of time.

MULTIPLE UNIVERSES AND SUPERIMPLICATE ORDERS:

Another of Bohm's propositions was that the implicate order contains within it all possibilities. The implicate order contains every subatomic particle that has ever been or ever will be as well as every possible configuration of matter and energy. The implicit order gives rise not to just one universe, but to many universes, to any number of explicate orders, parallel universes, and multiverses. He further hypothesized that the implicate order arises from the "superimplicate order," and that the superimplicate order arises from even deeper levels of reality.

196

HOLONS AND HOLARCHIES:

Arthur Koestler (1905-1983), an Hungarian-born author, philosopher, and professor, was truly a Renaissance man, whose ever-changing politics, career, and life led him to take up residence in a number of countries and to marry three times. His intellectual pursuits eventually culminated in attempting to use the theory of quantum physics to establish a scientific basis for extrasensory perception and Jung's synchronicity (1972; 1973). Koestler willed his estate to establish the position of Chair of Parapsychology at the Edinburgh University.

Among his many achievements, Koestler observed that every identifiable unit of organization, whether inorganic materials, biological organisms, or social organizations, consisted of smaller, more basic units, which were in turn comprised of even smaller units, and that every identifiable unit was part of a larger unit of organization. To describe the nature of these interconnections, Koestler proposed the word "holon," using the Greek word "holos," meaning "whole" and the suffix "on," meaning "part."

A "holon" is a whole that is part of another whole. More specifically, a "holon" is an identifiable part of a system or larger whole, it has its own unique identity, and it is made up of smaller, sub-ordinate parts. For example, an atom is a whole and is part of a molecule. A cell is a whole and is part of a body. A human is whole and is part of a society. A planet is a whole and is part of a solar system. A star is a whole and is part of a galaxy.

Koestler proposed that holons are organized into multilevel systems called "holarchies." The term "holarchy" is similar to the term "hierarchy." Besides including the Greek word "holos," the term "holarchy" was considered to be more appropriate because the term "hierarchy" has come to imply that higher levels are "better than" the lower levels and that the higher levels "control" or "have authority over" lower levels. Additionally, the term "hierarchy" is often associated with "paternal" and/or "male" dominance. In a holarchy, no one level is "better" or more valuable than any other level, and each holon acts independently of higher level holons, but is also able to receive instructions or guidance from higher level holons in the holarchy.

All holons behave or function in somewhat predictable ways or according to predictable laws. There are a number of forces or properties that are characteristic of all holons and holarchies. So far, approximately twenty such laws or characteristics of holons and holarchies have been identified.

For example, holons are said to emerge "holarchically." That is, wholes become parts of new wholes. The whole of one level becomes a part of the whole of the next level, establishing increased order and wholeness.

Several ways have been identified in which a holarchy or its holons may become pathological. In one such process, a holon may attempt to dominate the holarchy. In a multicellular organism, this situation is synonymous with the conditions referred to as cancerous. The ideal cure for this particular pathology is to integrate the holon back into its natural position in the holarchy.

HOLONS OF CONSCIOUSNESS AND INTEGRAL PSYCHOLOGY:

Wilbur (2000) proposed that psycho-spiritual growth in the individual human being occurs in progressive or holarchical levels of consciousness. He refers to these levels as "holons of consciousness." Each new level emerges from the previous level by disidentifying with it. Then each new level integrates the "structures" of the previous level in a holarchical pattern of increasing order and wholeness. Using the characteristics of holons and holarchies, Wilbur describes various healthy and pathological states that may occur at each new emerging level or "fulcrum" of development.

A book **"Through the Eyes of a Traveler"** by John Terry and Bonny Adams is fantastic. Maybe they are able to do what they are able to do because of 'just what we have been talking about.'

198

SECTION FIVE
Books that have greatly influenced me

As a Man Thinketh	James Allen
Celestine Prophecy	James Redfield
Creating Affluence	Deepak Chopra
Embraced by the Light	Betty Eadie
Gifts from A Course in Miracles	Frances Vaughan & Roger Walsh
Healing From the Heart	Judi Moore
Intention	Wayne Dyer
Les Miserables	Victor Hugo
Life in the World UNSEEN	Anthony Borgia
Laws of Success	Sterling W. Sill
Law of the Higher Potential	Robert Collier
Reprinted as "Riches within Your Reach"	
Miracle of Forgiveness	Spencer W. Kimbal
Mutant Message from Down Under	Marlo Morgan
Return from Tomorrow	George Ritchie
Return to Love	Marianne Williamson
Scriptures	Jesus Christ and his Prophets
Speaker for the Dead	Orson Scott Card
Through the Eyes of a Traveler	John Terry & Bonny Adams
Way of the Peaceful Warrior	Dan Millman
Your Sacred Self	Wayne Dyer

There are so many other great books that I have read and got much from. The most valued are the ones that teach mental and physical healing through unconditional love.

Again I emphasize, READ, READ, READ. If you come from a dysfunctional family as most people do from my experience, reading and dissolving issues thru inner energy work will bring unity to your inner being and your outer being. I am a witness to that.

My soul song is "Heal the World" by World Music Artists and close to that is "From a Distance" by Bette Midler and "Oh I believe there are angels among us." I make every effort to see the World and people from a distance at the same time I am yearning for the world to heal and I know God sends his Angels.

I do everything in my power to assist people to heal. The spirit within has a driving desire to be one with the human without. The ways I have mentioned in this book can assist in accomplishing this task.

I do not wish to offend any one just because of my honesty. Those of you who do not believe in God, that's O.K. That is your choice. It does not mean that He does not exist and it doesn't mean He doesn't love you anyway. He will be there for you in your time of need. If you need to experience something to assist you in growing more unified, He will allow you to make a mistake and learn from it.

See movie **"Peaceful Warrior"**

Some of
My Favorite Sayings and Thoughts
Sayings that have assisted me through the years:

Energy follows thought
Let Go and Let God
Gratitude attitude drowns pity and misery
There goes I but for the Grace of God
This too will Pass
Welcome failure. It is a stepping stone to success

I think most people are basically good so when someone does something offensive, I say something like "Out of Character."
By using that phrase, there have been people who have gone back to their true character.

The universe does not judge us; it only provides consequences and lessons and opportunities to balance and learn through the law of cause and effect.

Compassion is the recognition that we are each doing the best we can within the limits of our current beliefs and capacities

TIPS

1. Stuff a miniature marshmallow in the bottom of a sugar cone to prevent ice cream drips

2. Use a meat baster to "Squeeze" your pancake batter into the hot griddle- perfect shaped pancakes every time.

3. To keep potatoes from budding, place an apple in the bag with the potatoes.

4. To prevent egg shells from cracking, add a pinch of salt to the water before hard-boiling.

5. Use a pastry blender to cut ground beef into small pieces after browning.

6. For easy "Meatloaf mixing," combine the ingredients with a potato masher.

7. Run your hands under cold water before pressing Rice Krispies treats in the pan so the marshmallow won't stick to your fingers

8. Mash and freeze ripe bananas, in one-cup portions, for use in later baking, no wasted bananas (or you can freeze them whole, peeled, in plastic baggies)

9. To quickly use that frozen juice concentrate, simply mash it with a potato masher; no need to wait for it to thaw.

10. To get the most juice out of fresh lemons, bring them to room temperature and roll them under your palm against the kitchen counter before squeezing.

11. To easily remove burnt on food from your skillet, simply add a drop or two of dish soap and enough water to cover bottom of pan, and bring to a boil on stove-top. Skillet will be much easier to clean now, or just soak with dishwasher detergent and hot water. Then there is no need to boil

12. Spray your Tupperware with nonstick cooking spray before pouring in tomato-based sauces. No more stains.

13. Transfer your jelly to a small spastic squeeze bottle. No more mess, sticky jars or knives.

14. To aid in washing dishes, add a tablespoon of baking soda to your soapy water. It softens hands while cutting through grease.

15. When a cake recipe calls for flouring the baking pan, use a bit of the dry cake mix instead. No white mess on the outside of the cake.
16. If you accidentally over-salt a dish while it's still cooking, drop in a peeled potato. It absorbs the excess salt for an instant "fix me up."
17. Next time you need a quick ice pack, grab a bag of frozen vegetables out of your freezer. No watery leaks from a plastic baggie.
18. Rinse cooked, ground meat with water to wash away even more fat.
19. Wrap celery in aluminum foil when putting in the refrigerator. It will keep for weeks.
20. Substitute half applesauce for the vegetable oil in your baking recipes. You'll greatly reduce the fat content.
21. Brush beaten egg white over pie crust before baking to yield a beautiful glossy finish.
22. Place a slice of bread in hardened brown sugar to soften it back up.
23. When boiling corn on the cob, add a pinch of sugar to help bring out the corns natural sweetness
24. To determine whether an egg is fresh, immerse it in a pan of cool, salted water. If it sinks, it is fresh. If it rises to the surface, throw it away.
25. To clean a toilet. Drop in two Alka-Seltzer tablets, wait twenty minutes, brush and flush. The citric acid and effervescent action clean vitreous china.
26. To clean a vase. To remove a stain from the bottom of a glass vase or cruet, fill with water and drop in two Alka-Seltzer tablets.
27. Polish jewelry. Drop two Alka-Seltzer tablets into a glass of water and immerse the jewelry for two minutes.
28. Clean a thermos bottle by filling the bottle with water and drop in four Alka-Seltzer tablets and let soak for an hour or longer.
29. Unclog a drain by dropping three Alka-Seltzer tablets down the drain followed by a cup of White vinegar. Wait a few minutes and run the hot water.
30. Have a head ache? Take a lime, cut it in half and rub it on your forehead. The throbbing should go.

202

31.   If you have a problem opening jars, try using latex dishwashing gloves. They give a non-slip grip that makes opening jars easy.

32.   Potatoes will take food stains off fingers. Just slice and rub raw potato on the stains and rinse with water

33.   Methods to get rid of ants without the poison: Draw a chalk line on the floor, wall or wherever ants enter your house. Ants do not cross a chalk line. They also avoid nutmeg. Sprinkle it where the ants are coming in, and enjoy the smell.

34.   Mice hate catnip and cats love it. Plant it as close to the house as possible. Mice love valerian root. The Pied piper of Hamlin had Valerian Root in his bags. It wasn't the music that the mice liked. Plant it as far away from yours and your neighbor's house a possible. No more poison.

35.   Windows and mirrors clean up really good with air freshener and leave the room smelling wonderful.

36.   Splinters come out really well with scotch tape and it is painless and easy.

37.   Cover your body with olive oil or massage oil or other oils before showering and your skin should come out silky soft.

38.   Take a bath in Skin-So-Soft before you camp and bring some with you to keep the mosquito's way.

39.   Many uses for Bounce:
   a.   Bounce will chase ants away when you lay a sheet near them.
   b.   Bounce takes the odor out of books and photo albums that don't get opened too often.
   c.   Bounce repels mosquitoes. Tie a sheet of Bounce through a belt loop when outdoors during mosquito season.
   d.   Eliminate static electricity from your television screen. Wipe your television screen with a used sheet of Bounce to keep dust from resettling.
   e.   Dissolve soap scum from shower doors. Clean with a sheet of Bounce.
   f.   Freshen your home with Bounce

g. Prevent thread from tangling. Run a threaded needle through a sheet of Bounce before beginning to sew.

h. Prevent musty suitcases. Place an individual sheet of Bounce inside empty luggage before storing.

i. Freshen the air in your car. Place a sheet of Bounce under the front seat.

j. Clean baked-on foods from a cooking pan. Put a sheet in a pan, fill with water, let sit overnight, and sponge clean. It weakens the bond and soften the food.

k. Eliminate odors in wastebaskets or dirty laundry basket. Place a sheet of bounce at the bottom of the wastebasket or hamper

l. Wipe up sawdust from drilling or sand papering. A used sheet of Bounce will collect sawdust like a tack cloth.

m. Collect cat hair by rubbing Bounce. It will magnetically attract all the loose hairs.

n. Deodorize shoes or sneakers. Place a sheet of Bounce in your shoes or sneakers overnight so they will smell better in the morning.

o. Eliminate static electricity from Venetian blinds. Wipe the blinds with a sheet of Bounce to prevent dust from resettling.

Healing modalities that are Free

Some of them, to be literally free you will need to borrow, beg or barter. Or you may already have some supplies at home.

Modality	Supplies needed
Affirmation	Thoughts writing material Recording device
Art	Water, paint and paper
Breath	Concentration
Color	Crayons and paper
Dream	Thoughts
Exercise	A floor or bed
Laughter/Humor	Books/movies/friends
Rainbow	Thoughts
Script	Writing materials or use this book's script
Writing	Writing materials
Yoga	Yoga magazine or book

Healing modalities that cost about the same as you are spending already

This is not the case if you are getting food and medicine for free. If you are not, the following can save you money or at least assist you in breaking even and save a lot of time and poor health.

Quantum Energy: **Layers of Light** – the missing link: Oxygenated Water, Quantum Energy System
Nutritional: **Eniva,** Food State - Goji – Primal Cell Technology
Photo Therapy: PhotoMax
Weight Loss: Isagenix

Modalities where the initial investment is significant

In these cases the cost averages out pennies a day.

They are also the

Modalities that are easiest to use

Although the investment is significant, these are well worth investigating.

Nikken: Air Filter & in house water system, Infrared Products

Chi Machine – Passive exercise machine

FIR Hot House: Used in hospitals for chronic & critical patients

Products and how to obtain them

e-mail me at dianne_hoffmann@yahoo.com

Layers of Light www.2lolii.com/dandyone

e-mail for book no_one_thing@comcast.net

Centerpointe: Music for brain integration and Meditation

Eniva: VIBE Excellent nutritional in Physicians Desk Reference

Food State: Excellent nutritional

FreeLife: Goji juice. Excellent nutritional to cut down on sugar

HTE: Chi Machine & FIR Hot house (Dome) Exercise Plus

Isagenix: Great Weight Loss plan. Plus

Layers of Light Oxygenated Water. Quantum Energy System

Nikken: Magnetic and infrared products-,

NuSkin, Pharmanex, Big Planet, Photo Max: Skin Care +

Primal Cell Technologies: Makes the food you eat good for you.

Too good to be true? It is **true to be good!**

There are more Products that I can refer you to. There are too many to mention here.

Learning & Testing
Affirmations

I think clearly. My mental processes are sharp. I concentrate easily. Concentration is easy for me. I enjoy concentrating. I concentrate with ease. I am relaxed when I am concentrating. I feel at ease when I am concentrating. I feel joy as I concentrate. I am focused when I concentrate. I love concentrating. I concentrate with positive thought.

I have a powerful memory. Details are easy for me. Memory flows effortlessly. My powerful memory serves me well. My powerful memory makes me feel powerful. My cells exude powerful memory. My cells feel refreshed. As I use my powerful memory my powerful memory is strong and quick. I feel powerful as my quick accurate memory serves me. I remember all that is beneficial. I recall all the information I need whenever I need it. My memory serves me well. I have perfect memory and recall. I recall and retain what I need to know. I use my memory effortlessly. I focus easily. I read with comprehension. I listen intently. I am efficient with powerful memory. I am powerful in memory. I am quick to remember. I am powerful and quick with accurate memory. I exude powerful memory. I am excellent with details.

I believe in myself. I understand what I read. I am quick to answer correctly. I answer questions completely and correctly the first time. I enjoy reading. I clearly understand quickly as I read. My eyes focus for me as I read. My eyes see clearly as I read. I am wide awake and alert as I read. My eyes are relaxed while I read. My eyes serve me well. I can see clearly as I read and understand what I read. Reading is fun. I learn as I read. I enjoy learning as I read. Reading is enjoyable. I love to understand what I read. I feel powerful as I read. I am powerful when I read. I feel great energy surge through me as I understand what I read. I retain all of what I read. I am alert. I am quick. I am a genius. I am intuitive. My mind is keen. I am insightful. I am positive. I can read anything that is beneficial to me. I am academically successful.

I am positive. I can do anything. I am a winner. I think positively. I expect only the best in my academic endeavors. I am a clear thinker. I choose the best pathway for the best outcome. I am awake. I am aware. I am alert. I am confident. I am focused. I am always recognizing that which is for my highest good.

I am smart. I excel at tests. I enjoy tests. I remember easily. I am relaxed during tests. Answers come to me easily. I am relaxed and confident as I take tests. Information flows through me.
I am alert. I am quick. I am a genius. I am intuitive. I dream solutions. My mind is keen. I am insightful.

I am good at math. Math is effortless. I think logically. I am excellent in logic. My logic is excellent. I quickly see successful solutions to problems. I am logical. Math is simple. I enjoy figuring out math problems quickly and accurately. I am relaxed as I figure out the solution to the math problem. I am confident in my ability to solve the math problem. I am positive. I can learn and understand any math given me. I solve problems easily. I enjoy solving problems. I solve math problems easily. I enjoy solving math problems quickly.

I imagine with all my senses. Stimuli are sensory rich. I solve problems easily. I enjoy solving problems easily. I am relaxed as I solve problems.

I have a powerful vocabulary. I use words correctly. I speak well. I write well. I spell well. I am articulate. I enjoy speaking. I am a powerful speaker. I love to speak. I am a clear thinker. I see the whole picture. I am good with words. I express myself well. People understand me as I speak with confidence. I am a powerful speaker My mind is keen. I am alert. I am quick. I am a genius. I am a positive speaker. I am energetic as I speak. I am confident as I listen. I understand as others speak. I enjoy listening to others alternate views. I am able to use what I hear to benefit myself and others. My mind is powerful. I can do, say and write successfully. I am a success in speaking. I am a success in writing. I am a success in remembering. I am a success in action. My words are positive. My words are inspiring. I am positive. I am a success. I am powerful. I am inspiring. I choose success in speaking. I choose success in writing. I believe in myself. I am creative in speaking. I am creative in writing. I am creative in doing. I am creative in thinking. I feel myself being creative and ingenious. My present and future are filled with creative thought, words and actions.

I have a powerful memory. Details are easy. Memory flows effortlessly. My powerful memory is constant. I think clearly. My mental processes are sharp. I am powerful. I am smart. I am quick. I am a genius. I am a keen thinker. I am focused. I am powerful. I am energetic. I am relaxed.

Prosperity & Abundance Affirmations

I think clearly. My mental processes are sharp. I concentrate easily. Concentration is easy for me. I enjoy concentrating. I concentrate with ease. I am relaxed when I am concentrating. I feel at ease when I am concentrating. I feel joy as I concentrate. I am focused when I concentrate. I love concentrating. I concentrate with positive thought.

I have a powerful memory. Details are easy for me. Memory flows effortlessly. My powerful memory serves me well. My powerful memory makes me feel powerful. My cells exude powerful memory. My cells feel refreshed. As I use my powerful memory my powerful memory is strong and quick. I feel powerful as my quick accurate memory serves me. I remember all that is beneficial. I recall all the information I need whenever I need it. My memory serves me well. I have perfect memory and recall. I recall and retain what I need to know. I use my memory effortlessly. I focus easily. I read with comprehension. I listen intently. I am efficient with powerful memory. I am powerful in memory. I am quick to remember. I am powerful and quick with accurate memory. I exude powerful memory. I am excellent with details.

I believe in myself. I understand what I read. I am quick to answer correctly. I answer questions completely and correctly the first time. I enjoy reading. I clearly understand quickly as I read. My eyes focus for me as I read. My eyes see clearly as I read. I am wide awake and alert as I read. My eyes are relaxed while I read. My eyes serve me well. I can see clearly as I read and understand what I read. Reading is fun. I learn as I read. I enjoy learning as I read. Reading is enjoyable. I love to understand what I read. I feel powerful as I read. I am powerful when I read. I feel great energy surge through me as I understand what I read. I retain all of what I read. I am alert. I am quick. I am a genius. I am intuitive. My mind is keen. I am insightful. I am positive. I can read anything that is beneficial to me. I am academically successful.

I am positive. I can do anything. I am a winner. I think positively. I expect only the best in my academic endeavors. I am a clear thinker. I choose the best pathway for the best outcome. I am awake. I am aware. I am alert. I am confident. I am focused. I am always recognizing that which is for my highest good. I am alert. I am quick. I am a genius. I am intuitive. I dream solutions. My mind is keen. I am insightful. I imagine with all my senses. Stimuli are sensory rich. I solve easily. I enjoy solving problems easily. I am relaxed as I solve problems.

I have a powerful vocabulary. I use words correctly. I speak well. I write well. I spell well. I am articulate. I enjoy speaking. I am a powerful speaker. I love to speak I am a clear thinker. I see the whole picture. I am good with words. I express myself well. People understand me as I speak with confidence. I am a powerful speaker. My mind is keen. I am alert. I am quick. I am a genius. I am a positive speaker. I am energetic as I speak. I am confident as I listen. I understand as others speak. I enjoy listening to others alternate views. I am able to use what I hear to benefit myself and others. My mind is powerful. I can do, say or rite successfully. I am a success in speaking. I am a success in writing. I am a success in remembering. I am a success in actions. My words are positive. My words are inspiring. I am positive. I am a success. I am powerful. I am inspiring. I choose success in speaking. I choose success in writing. I believe in myself. I am creative in speaking. I am creative in writing. I am creative in doing. I am creative in thinking. I feel myself being creative and ingenious. My present and my future are filled with creative thought, words and actions.

I have a powerful memory. Details are easy. Memory flows effortlessly. My powerful memory is constant. I think clearly. My mental processes are sharp. I am powerful. I am energetic. I am relaxed. I am powerful. I feel great. Energy surges through me. I am abundantly energetic. Life is fantastic. I am filled with energy. I am relaxed. I am calm. I am in control. I am at peace with myself. I am at peace with the world. I stand erect. I sit erect. I am confident. My body parts work in perfect harmony. I move with my head up and my shoulders back. I am proud of my body. I feel the presence and power of motivation. I am empowered by the energy and thought of good health. I love my work. My work helps to keep me healthy. I am productive. I see the purpose of each task necessary to keep me healthy and fit. I understand the importance of work for my health. I see the importance of exercise for my health. I understand the importance of good eating habits for my health. I believe in myself. I am focused on my goal of health. I am focused on my goal of fitness. I am attuned to my goal of health. I am attuned to my goal of fitness. I am focused on exercise. I am intuitive to good foods for my body. I release all thought of unhealthy food. My body knows the food best for my body.

I have good vision. I exercise my eyes. I care for my eyes. My eyes are healthy. My eyes are focused. Images are clear. My eyes focus, I can see clearly. I stand erect. I sit erect. I move with my head up and my shoulders back. I am proud of my body. I nurture my body with positive thought. I am strong and vital. I chose to be thin I achieve the perfect weight for my healthy body. I am powerful. I feel great. Energy surges

210

through me. I am abundantly energetic. Life is fantastic. I choose health. Exercise is fun. I care for myself. I exercise regularly. I love exercising. I breathe deeply. I am relaxed. I am calm. I am in control. I am at peace with myself. I am at peace with the world. I feel young. My cells are young and healthy. I look young. My body is strong. My skin radiates youth and health. My skin is young. My skin is clear. My skin is healthy. My skin is vibrant. I care for my body. I am healthy. I eat properly.

I am safe. I am at peace. I am worthwhile. I love and approve of myself. I am loving and lovable. I am a divine expression of life. I love and accept myself where I am right now. I choose to love and enjoy myself. I lovingly take care of my body. I lovingly take care of my mind. I lovingly take care of my emotions. I love and approve of myself. I am important. I am powerful and capable of creating and maintaining a perfect body. I chose to see my self-worth. I love and approve of my self. I am a beautiful expression of life. I experience joy in my healthy body. I love life. I love and approve of myself. I am willing to experience life. I am safe. I choose to see with love I am cherished and loved. I know that life always supports me. I am free to move forward with love in my heart.

I experience my intuition as a loving trusted friend. My intuition guides me to my highest good. I am awake and aware. I recall all the information I need whenever I need it. My memory serves me well. I have perfect memory and recall. I recall and retain what I need to know. I use my memory effortlessly. I believe in myself. I believe in my products. My sales benefit me and serve others. I see myself successfully selling. I overcome objections with ease. I am a strong closer. I am persuasive and successful. I love my work. I am productive. I see the purpose of each task clearly. I perform challenging tasks with energy and focus. I can handle all that I receive. I am moved to act by thought. I feel the presence of power of motivation. I am empowered by the energy and thought of creativity.

I am a clear thinker I am a decision maker. I see the whole picture. I listen for the sound of possibilities. I choose the best pathway for the best outcome. I know the source of my infinite supply. I am rich in thought, word and deed. I am blessed beyond my wildest dreams. My prosperity benefits others. I create the income I desire. I feel myself being creative and ingenious. Creativity flows to and through me. My present and my future are filled with creative thoughts, words and actions. I believe in myself. I release all thoughts and relationships that no longer serve my highest good. I am focused and attuned to my goals. I trust myself. I am a winner.

Health & Fitness
Affirmations

I have good vision. I exercise my eyes. I care for my eyes. My eyes are healthy. My eyes are focused. Images are clear. My eyes focus. I can see clearly. I enjoy eating foods that assist my eyes to see perfectly. I enjoy seeing perfectly. I appreciate my perfect eye sight. My eyes feel great. My eyes see great. My eyes see clearly. My eyes see perfectly. The nerves in my eyes are healthy. I have a perfect brain. I have a healthy brain. My eyes feel great. My eyes are relaxed. My eyes see effortlessly. I am excellent at seeing. I am successful at seeing clearly. All my cells work together for the good of my eyesight. I enjoy seeing clearly. I am focused on perfect eyesight. I accept perfect eye sight. I am joyous of perfect eyesight.

I am powerful. I feel great. Energy surges through me. I am abundantly energetic. Life is fantastic. I am filled with energy. My cells remember and produce health. I am focused on health. I accept perfect health. My body is perfect. I am healthy. I choose health. Exercise is fun. I care for myself. I exercise regularly. I love exercising. I breathe deeply. I eat the right foods. My body burns off fat. My body is efficient. I am energetic. I treat myself well. I am Healthy. I am loved. I love other people. I am safe. I am relaxed. I am calm. I am in control. I am at peace with myself. I am at peace with the world. I stand erect. I sit erect. I am confident. My body parts work in perfect harmony. I move with my head up and my shoulders back. I am proud of my body. I nurture my body with positive thought I am strong and vital. I choose to be thin. I am thin. I choose to be trim. I am trim. I choose to be physically fit. I am physically fit. I achieve the perfect weight for my healthy body. My body dissolves fat continually. I feel young. My cells are young and healthy. I look young. My body is strong. My skin radiates youth and health. My skin is young I am young. My skin is clear I am clear. My skin is healthy. I am healthy. My skin is vibrant. I am vibrant. I care for my body. I eat properly.

I feel the presence and power of motivation. I am empowered by the energy and thought of good health. I love my work. My work helps to keep me healthy. I am productive. I see the purpose of each task necessary to keep me healthy and fit. I understand the importance of work for my health. I see the importance of exercise for my health. I understand the importance of good eating habits for my health. I believe in myself. I am focused on my goal of health. I am focused on my goal of fitness. I am attuned to my goal of health. I am attuned to my goal of fitness. I am

212

focused on exercise. I am intuitive to good foods for my body. I release all thought of unhealthy food. My body knows the food best for my body.

I have good vision. I exercise my eyes. I care for my eyes. My eyes are healthy. My eyes are focused. Images are clear. My eyes focus. I can see clearly. My cells remember and produce health. I am focused on health. I enjoy optimal health. I accept perfect health. My body is perfect. I am healthy. I eat the right foods. My body burns off fat. My body is efficient. I am energetic. I am proud of my body. I nurture my body with positive thoughts. I am strong and vital. I choose to be thin. I achieve the perfect weight for my healthy body. I am powerful. I feel great. Energy surges through me. I am abundantly energetic. Life is fantastic. I choose health. Exercise is fun. I care for myself. I exercise regularly. I love exercising. I breathe deeply. I am relaxed. I am calm. I am in control. I am at peace with myself. I am at peace with the world. I feel young. My cells are young and healthy. I look young. My body is strong. My skin radiates youth and health. My skin is young. My skin is clear. My skin is healthy. My skin is vibrant. I care for my body. I am healthy. I eat properly.

I am safe. I am at peace. I am worthwhile. I love and approve of myself. I am loving and lovable. I am a divine expression of life. I love and accept myself where I am right now. I choose to love and enjoy myself. I lovingly take care of my body. I lovingly take care of my mind. I lovingly take care of my emotions. I love and approve of myself. I am important. I am powerful and capable of creating and maintaining a perfect body. I choose to see my self-worth. I love and approve of myself. I am a beautiful expression of life. I experience joy in my healthy body. I love life. I love and approve of myself. I am willing to experience life. I am safe. I choose to see with love. I am cherished and loved I know that life always supports me. I am free to move forward with love in my heart. I believe in myself. I release all thought and relationships that no longer serve my highest good. I am focused and attuned to my goals. I trust myself. I am a winner.

Index

Upcoming Events
Look for more No One Thing™ books to come
No One Thing™ Retreat

Printed in the United States
83840LV00002B/172-393/A